Cannabis Extracts
in Medicine

McFarland Health Topics Series

CANNABIS EXTRACTS IN MEDICINE

The Promise of Benefits in Seizure Disorders, Cancer and Other Conditions

Jeffrey Dach, M.D.,
Elaine A. Moore *and*
Justin Kander

MCFARLAND HEALTH TOPICS

McFarland & Company, Inc., Publishers
Jefferson, North Carolina

ALSO BY ELAINE A. MOORE: *The Amphetamine Debate: The Use of Adderall, Ritalin and Related Drugs for Behavior Modification, Neuroenhancement and Anti-Aging Purposes* (2011) • *Hepatitis: Causes, Treatments and Resources* (2006) • *Autoimmune Diseases and Their Environmental Triggers* (2002)

BY ELAINE A. MOORE AND LISA MOORE: *Advances in Graves' Disease and Other Hyperthyroid Disorders* (2013) • *Encyclopedia of Alzheimer's Disease; With Directories of Research, Treatment and Care Facilities*, 2d ed. (2012) • *Encyclopedia of Sexually Transmitted Diseases* (2005; paperback 2009) • *Graves' Disease: A Practical Guide* (2001)

BY ELAINE A. MOORE AND SAMANTHA WILKINSON: *The Promise of Low Dose Naltrexone Therapy: Potential Benefits in Cancer, Autoimmune, Neurological and Infectious Disorders* (2009)

ALL FROM MCFARLAND

This book is an educational resource and is not meant as a substitute for professional medical advice. Individuals interested in the use of cannabis extracts should consult a medical practitioner with experience using cannabis extracts.

LIBRARY OF CONGRESS CATALOGUING-IN-PUBLICATION DATA

Dach, Jeffrey, 1950– , author.
    Cannabis extracts in medicine : the promise of benefits in seizure disorders, cancer, and other conditions / Jeffrey Dach, Elaine A. Moore, and Justin Kander.
        p. cm. — (McFarland health topics)
    Includes bibliographical references and index.

    ISBN 978-0-7864-9663-1 (softcover : acid free paper) ∞
    ISBN 978-1-4766-2111-1 (ebook)

    I. Moore, Elaine A., 1948– , author. II. Kander, Justin, 1991– , author. III. Title. IV. Series: McFarland health topics.
[DNLM: 1. Cannabinoids—therapeutic use. 2. Medical Marijuana—therapeutic use. 3. Neoplasms—drug therapy. 4. Seizures—drug therapy. QV 77.7]
    RM666.C266
    615.3'2345—dc23   2015027520

BRITISH LIBRARY CATALOGUING DATA ARE AVAILABLE

Front cover images © 2015 iStock/Thinkstock

Printed in the United States of America

McFarland & Company, Inc., Publishers
  Box 611, Jefferson, North Carolina 28640
    www.mcfarlandpub.com

To patients with seizure disorders and cancer
who remain untreated or imprisoned due to
their inability to legally obtain cannabis extracts;
and to the many researchers who are investigating
the full individual uses of cannabis extracts.

Acknowledgments

Jeff would like to express his gratitude to his wife, Judith, and their children, Ari, Benjamin, and Karina, for their help and support while he worked on this project.

Elaine would especially like to thank her son Brett for giving her the idea to write this book after learning about Charlotte Figi's use of cannabidiol for her seizure disorders in local news reports. Knowing of his mother's experience with alternative medicine and in toxicology, specifically with NIDA drug testing, he saw this as a perfect fit. She'd also like to thank Sammy Jo Wilkinson for sharing her successful use of cannabidiol for MS and her husband, Doug Flomer, for providing us with images of the cannabis oil extraction process. Credit is also due to Martin Lee, Michelle Sexton, Dustin Sulak, Jason Marhu, and Valerie Corral for their comprehensive online course on cannabidiol and its medical uses in July and August 2014. Their willingness to answer questions is greatly appreciated. Elaine would also like to thank her niece Carrie Pacer for her work compiling our resource chapter. Rick Moore, Lisa Moore, and Judy Canfield vigilantly watched all news sources so that Elaine could keep up with the rapid changes in the cannabis playing field. The librarians at the New York Public Library District have been an invaluable resource. Elaine would also like to thank her friends Trish Hill and Ben Coe for their expertise in cultivars and Ascha Karen Champie for introducing the authors to Christopher Larson. Last but not least, she'd like to thank Dave Mapes from Epsilonresearch.org for his generous sharing of information and images.

Justin is very thankful to Students for Sensible Drug Policy for all the magical ways they have facilitated his development. He's also grateful to Aunt Zelda's, Patients Out of Time, the Phoenix Tears Foundation, United Patients Group, Sirius Extracts, and Illegally Healed.

Table of Contents

Introduction
by Elaine A. Moore

As 2013 neared its end, cannabis dominated the news in Colorado. Recreational sales of cannabis were about to begin, and for the first time in nearly 80 years, cannabis could be sold for general use. However, the far more important news story involved a young girl named Charlotte Figi and how a specific type of cannabis extract changed her life.

The cannabis oil Charlotte's physician used to successfully treat her intractable seizure disorder is high in cannabidiol (CBD), a component of cannabis with medicinal but not psychoactive properties. This particular oil was primarily derived from a hybrid strain (cannabis and industrial hemp) called Charlotte's Web, developed by the Stanley Brothers in Colorado. This strain was originally designed to stop cancer metastasis but was redirected towards epilepsy after reports of CBD's effectiveness in seizure disorders was described by researchers in California. The Stanley Brothers and the Figi family have been instrumental in broadcasting Charlotte's story. They made their debut in 2012 on the National Geographic series *American Weed*. Later, they achieved greater prominence through a CNN special called *Weed*, hosted by Dr. Sanjay Gupta, which examined their work alongside other cannabis-related news.

Substantial research is currently being undertaken to investigate the medical benefits of CBD, and the existing research is already very promising. In particular, researchers are examining cannabinoid receptors, interactions between endocannabinoids and phytocannabinoids, and especially the role of CBD in seizure disorders, head trauma, post–traumatic stress disorder, chronic neuropathic pain, cancer, and psychiatric disorders. For instance, a November 2013 report on laboratory, ani-

1

mal, and preclinical studies issued by the National Cancer Institute shows that CBD has chemoprotective properties in breast and colon cancer.

Mainstream news and scientific sources are reporting human success stories, including an infant treated successfully for brain cancer with a CBD-rich extract, a UK patient who treated himself successfully for terminal liver cancer, and a patient beating an aggressive optic pathway glioma. Further reports include an infant successfully treated with CBD for glioblastoma, a patient in the UK successfully treated for colon cancer, and patients in remission from breast cancer. It's hardly surprising that on September 29, 2014, Insys Therapeutics announced that the United States Food and Drug Administration had granted orphan drug designation to its proprietary cannabidiol product for the treatment of glioma.

For advocates of medical marijuana and botanists, these reports aren't surprising. Plants have a variety of chemicals that can induce physiological effects within the body. The plant foxglove is used to make the heart medicine digitalis. Willow bark yields acetylsalicylic acid (aspirin). Many of the pharmaceutical compounds synthesized in laboratories are designed to mimic the action of various plant derivatives. Since the year 5 BC, cannabis has been listed in the *Materia Medica* for its healing properties. While the hemp plant *Cannabis sativa* is more widely known for the psychoactive properties related to delta–9-tetrahydrocannabinol (THC), there's more to this plant. The various phytochemicals found in cannabis, especially CBD, have their own unique properties.

Since we first began writing this book in 2012, researchers have made major advances in cannabis research. Despite federal restrictions on research in the United States, experts worldwide are working together to share their findings. On November 21, 2014, co-author Justin Kander presented at the Inaugural Australian Medicinal Cannabis Symposium in Tamworth, Australia, about cannabis extracts for treating cancer. The event was attended by major politicians and news media, including Mike Baird, the premier of New South Wales. Other speakers included Dr. Lester Grinspoon, Dr. Ilya Reznik, Dr. Robert Melamede, and Australian law enforcement personnel, who together discussed the scientific and ethical rationale for ending medicinal cannabis prohibition. In July and August 2014, Martin Lee hosted an extensive online course on the use of CBD in current medical practices. The field is expanding at a rapid pace, and our goal is to keep the reader up to date on these advances.

Our book focuses on the biochemical properties, medical benefits, and physiological effects of CBD and other cannabinoids found in the cannabis plant. We've also presented views on the uses of industrial hemp as compared to CBD-rich cannabis strains, the reasons behind cannabis's Schedule I status, and an overview of current research, animal studies, anecdotal reports, and clinical trial reports. To explain how cannabis exerts its healing properties, we've described the ways in which CBD and other cannabinoids interact with the endocannabinoid system and modulate the immune system. This book is not meant as medical or treatment advice. Individuals, however, have a right to learn of all available treatment options. As with all our books, our goal in writing this book is to educate and empower patients.

ONE

Cannabidiol (CBD)

The *Cannabis sativa* L. plant contains more than 750 natural chemical compounds, including more than 100 unique cannabinoids (American Herbal Pharmacopoeia, 33). The two most abundant components of cannabis are the cannabinoids delta–9-tetrahydrocannabinol (THC) and cannabidiol (CBD). In recent years, studies have shown that these compounds have astonishing therapeutic value. Administered together, they create synergistic effects. The serendipitous 2009 discovery in California of CBD-rich strains, which have been used successfully to treat children with tumors and seizure disorders, has opened doors to what's become a patient-directed movement. Chapter One introduces readers to the cannabinoid known as cannabidiol, its physiological effects, and its escalating role as a medical therapy.

What Is Cannabidiol (CBD)?

The phytochemical cannabidiol has astonishing therapeutic potential, but unlike THC, CBD is devoid of psychoactive properties and therefore does not cause a "high." CBD has potent anti-inflammatory, antioxidant, anti-seizure, anti-rheumatic, anti-tumor, anti-anxiety, anti-emetic, and anti-bacterial properties. With mild sedating properties, CBD helps to reduce the psychoactive effects of THC in strains containing both cannabinoids.

As the second most prominent component in cannabis, CBD occurs in negligible to minimal amounts in popular recreational strains. The presence of cannabinoid receptors in the brain, peripheral nervous system, and immune system indicates (see Chapter Three) that the body is able to respond physiologically to the presence of CBD and other phytochem-

5

icals present in cannabis as well as naturally occurring (endogenous) cannabinoids. In light of this proven physiological response, the cannabis plant causes a variety of specific biological effects.

The CBD:THC Ratio

Under normal growing conditions, the flowers and resin of the cannabis plant contain far more THC than CBD. In fact, marijuana sold for recreational use in Colorado has very little CBD, typically .02 percent or less, although THC levels may be as high as 24 percent. Recreational cannabis typically is bred to have larger amounts of THC with almost no CBD to maximize psychoactivity. Both THC and CBD have a variety of therapeutic benefits, and their relative proportions in extracts are important for optimizing medicinal use. Plant extracts rich in CBD, for instance, have a number of documented medical uses, as do extracts with high THC content and smaller amounts of CBD. Medical marijuana dispensaries help clients find the strain types recommended by their physicians.

For example, in a presentation at the 2007 International Association of Cannabis as Medicine conference, Dr. Raphael Mechoulam, who first discovered THC and elucidated the chemical structure of CBD, described a small study conducted by Paul Consroe in which CBD was tested as a treatment for intractable epilepsy. In this study, patients stayed on the anticonvulsant medications they had been on (which failed to eliminate their seizures) and added 200 mg/day of CBD or a placebo. Of the seven patients getting CBD over the course of several months, only one showed no improvement. Three subjects became seizure-free, one experienced only one or two seizures over the course of the study, and two experienced reduced severity and occurrence of seizures, Mechoulam recalled (Mechoulam, "Mechoulam: On Cannabidiol," 1–2).

This report prompted growers in states where medical marijuana is legal to develop strains with increased CBD content. Depending on the ratio of CBD to THC in a particular plant strain or cultivar, cannabis derivatives can have different therapeutic effects. These effects can vary among different individuals, even those with the same disorders, but knowing what generally works well for others is a great foundation for any new patient to start with.

Other phytochemicals found in cannabis, such as fatty acids and aromatic terpenes, have also been investigated and have been found to have therapeutic benefits, leading some scientists to advocate using the entire plant as therapy (Frankel, 1). The properties and effects of the other phytochemicals in cannabis are described in Chapters Two and Five. The star cannabinoid making headlines, however, is CBD.

The Success of Cannabidiol

There is nothing inherently novel about CBD that pushed this cannabinoid into the limelight. What is new are increasing numbers of scientific studies and anecdotal success stories describing medicinal effects of CBD, especially benefits seen in children with seizure disorders and patients with multiple sclerosis (MS) and cancer. Early reports have inspired more researchers worldwide to conduct studies on CBD and other cannabinoids. A September 2014 search on PubMed, the National Library of Medicine search engine, for "cannabidiol" listed 1,248 separate journal articles.

CBD Research

While the medicinal benefits of cannabis have been reported for centuries, government policies have prevented adequate research into CBD's properties since it was first isolated from cannabis by Adams and Todd at the University of Illinois in 1940 (Zuardi). CBD studies, while scant in the 1950s and 1960s, peaked in the 1970s after Raphael Mechoulam and Yuval Shvo, chemists at the Daniel Sieff Research Institute Division of the Weizmann Institute of Science in Rehovoth, Israel, elucidated its chemical structure in 1963 (Mechoulam and Shvo, 1963).

Unfortunately, research on CBD soon faded in the 1980s, primarily due to federal government restrictions, sparse funding, political pressures, and a lack of interest in plants compared to the rapidly expanding world of synthetic pharmaceuticals. The Controlled Substances Act (CSA), enacted as Title II of the Comprehensive Drug Abuse Prevention and Control Act of 1970, which, against the advice of the American Medical Association (Kuipers, 117) classified cannabis as a Schedule I Drug, effectively put a halt to most of the ongoing CBD research just as the early reports of its medicinal effects were being discovered. Schedule I drugs are substances with no medical value and high potential for abuse. Schedule II drugs are seen as equally dangerous and include drugs like cocaine and methamphetamine, but because they have a defined medical use, they are still available by prescription. Drugs classified as Schedule I cannot be prescribed, and research into their medical benefits is substantially restricted.

The discovery of the endocannabinoid receptor system in 1992 (see Chapter Three) excited researchers and led to further CBD studies. With the knowledge that the body produces its own endogenous cannabinoids, researchers began investigating the ways in which both endocannabinoids and plant cannabinoids work to promote health. Patients have also helped tremendously in bringing CBD to the forefront. In recent years, anecdotal reports of CBD's success in treating seizure disorders (Gardner, "Realm of Caring") and cancer have accelerated research into its uses (Bunam, 1). More information on the medical uses of CBD can be found in Chapters Six and Seven. Recent and ongoing research studies and clinical trials are described in Chapter Eight.

Safety and Side Effects of CBD

While more studies are still needed, Bergamaschi and colleagues in Brazil conducted a systematic review of the medical literature, including human and animal studies, to assess the safety of CBD. Several studies suggested that CBD is non-toxic even in doses as high as 1500 mg/day and does not cause changes in appetite (as THC does), does not induce catalepsy (trance-like state without movement changes), does not affect vital signs (heart rate, blood pressure, and body temperature), and does not impair digestion, psychomotor, or psychological functions (Bergamaschi et al., 237–9).

Several studies that were evaluated in this review described a few potential side effects of cannabidiol. Of greatest significance, CBD inhibits hepatic drug metabolism, which can cause the co-administration of other drugs, including THC, to acquire increased potency. Alterations of cell viability in vitro (test tube studies) and slightly decreased fertilization capacity have also been noted. Based on recent advances in cannabinoid administration in humans, controlled CBD may be considered safe, but further studies are warranted (Bergamaschi et al., 238–40). In a recent online course focusing on the medical health revolution relating to CBD, Dustin Sulak, DO, reports that he has not seen many side effects reported in the hundreds of patients he treats with cannabinoid extracts. He reports that low CBD doses tend to have a stimulating effect, whereas high doses are sedating. Martin Lee, co-founder of Project CBD, made a similar observation and discussed this biphasic effect, explaining that CBD binds with the same adenosine receptors as caffeine. CBD may also block the increased appetite attributed to THC when cannabis strains with a high CBD:THC ratio are used (Lee and Sulak). THC also has a notable biphasic effect, in which low doses can alleviate anxiety but high doses often promote it.

From a historical view, CBD was common in cannabis landraces (a natural cannabis strain growing wild in a specific geographic area) from Afghanistan and Morocco, along with other countries. Because it lacks psychoactive properties, over the last hundred years it has largely been bred out of recreational cannabis. While CBD is present in hemp fiber and seed strains, it is usually found in low concentrations (Russo, "Cannabis Strains").

Cannabidivarin (CBDV)

A discussion of CBD cannot be complete without mentioning other cannabis components with therapeutic benefits, including the precursor acids of both THC and CBD (THCA and CBDA). Another cannabinoid under investigation, cannabidivarin (CBDV), is being used as a therapy for seizure disorders. CBDV and other cannabis phytochemicals are discussed further in Chapter Five.

Ancient Medicine

For nearly 5,000 years, the medicinal effects of cannabis have been well described, although the mechanisms responsible for these actions were unknown until recently (Goodman and Gilman, 2nd ed., 170). Just as these benefits were being discovered, they were simultaneously disregarded in the 20th century due to laws prohibiting the use of cannabis.

All of the medical benefits of cannabis, which were first described in China in 2737 BC and later confirmed in India, Egypt, and Europe (Goodman and Gilman, 2nd ed., 170), became part of ancient history. Many reports on the success of cannabis as a surgical anesthetic and for treating pain, dysentery, cholera, rheumatic diseases, and childbirth disorders (McMeens, 140) became irrelevant as the war to keep hemp from the public (see Chapter Nine) became a greater fight than the War on Drugs.

Later Research

In the early nineteenth century, university researchers first began to actively study the cannabis plant and its constituents. Until 1937, the growth and use of marijuana was legal under federal law. Unfortunately, cannabis studies were soon curtailed with the passage of the Marihuana Tax Act (MTA) of 1937, which unofficially banned the use of cannabis and ultimately led to the removal of cannabis from the U.S. Pharmacopoeia by 1942 (Grinspoon, "Cannabinopathic"). The MTA imposed a strict regulation requiring a high-cost transfer-tax stamp for every sale of cannabis. These stamps were rarely issued by the federal government.

Between 1854 and 1941, Parke-Davis, Eli Lilly, and Bristol-Meyers Squibb all produced cannabis extracts containing 60 mg of the drug in 0.5-ml formulas. These were used for a wide range of medical conditions, including headache, arthritis, neurological syndromes, insomnia, neuralgia, gonorrhea, and childbirth complications (Goodman and Gilman, 2nd ed., 175; McMeens, 129–30). Cannabis extracts and tinctures were also available in the UK and listed in the British Pharmacopoeia for more than 100 years (Amar). Great Britain and most European countries banned cannabis in the 1970s by adopting recommendations from the 1971 Convention on Psychotropic Substances instituted by the United Nations (Amar, 2).

The Success of CBD

Since both THC and CBD are highly lipid-soluble, they readily cross the blood-brain barrier and access the central nervous system. In 2014, William Courtney, MD, reported on an eight-month-old with a large brain tumor that was successfully treated with CBD in 2012 (Torres). In describing this achievement, Dr. Courtney emphasized the safety profile of CBD. He has also discussed how research conducted in Bethesda, Maryland, led to patent 6,630,507, which has been held by the United States of America since 2003. This patent demonstrates the antioxidant and neuroprotective effects of CBD and that lack of psychoactivity in CBD allows doses that are 100–200 times greater than the tolerable dose of THC (Courtney).

According to Dr. Courtney, cannabinoids can prevent cancer, reduce heart attacks by 66 percent, and reduce insulin-dependent diabetes by 58 percent. Dr. Courtney recommends drinking four to eight ounces of raw flower and leaf juice from any cannabis plant, 5 mg of CBD per kg of body weight, a salad of cannabis seed sprouts, and 50 mg of THC taken in 5 daily doses (Torres). The safety and benefits of CBD are also emphasized in a journal article from the UK that describes how CBD inhibits glioma cell migration in humans (Vaccani et al., 1032–3).

CBD Reduces Anxiety

CBD has anxiolytic (anxiety-reducing) properties (Campos et. al., "Cannabidiol Blocks," 1501–2); Zuardi and Guimarães, 134–6), which block the anxiogenic (anxiety-invoking) effects of THC. Studies show that in cannabis plants with a higher CBD:THC ratio, CBD can attenuate the psychoactive and anxiogenic effects of THC. Neuroimaging studies show that CBD changes brain activity related to emotional processing due to its interaction with the endocannabinoid system, effectively reducing the effects of post–traumatic stress disorder (PTSD). Besides its benefits in PTSD, CBD is also being studied in hepatic encephalopathy and in stroke (Campos et al., "Multiple Mechanisms").

Zuardi and Guimarães have found that when CBD is administered before THC, it potentiates the psychoactive effects of THC, probably due to a pharmacokinetic interaction. CBD is a potent inhibitor of the liver's drug-metabolizing enzymes (Joy, Watson, and Benson, 36). Therefore, in the presence of CBD, the concentrations of THC that reach the brain are higher than usual. However, when the two compounds are administered together, CBD antagonizes the psychoactive effects of THC. In the cannabis plant itself, CBD works to temper the effects of THC. Similarly, because psychosis can manifest with high doses of THC, CBD has the potential to reduce these effects. CBD has been shown to have anxiolytic and possibly antipsychotic effects (Zuardi and Guimarães, 136).

Early CBD Studies

In the first 45 years following the discovery of its chemical structure, several insights were discovered about CBD. It soon became apparent that the compound did not have the same psychoactive effects as THC. Together with THC, CBD was shown to have antiepileptic, anti-spasmodic, and sedative properties. During the 1980s and 1990s, CBD studies focused on its

11

anxiolytic, antipsychotic, and antispasmodic effects (Zuardi and Guimãres 1997, 136–9). In addition, early studies showed improvement in patients with spinal cord injuries using an extract containing THC, CBD, or a combination of the two cannabinoids administered as a sublingual spray (Amar, 15).

Later CBD Studies

In the last decade, further research has demonstrated CBD's therapeutic benefits in conditions such as Parkinson's disease, Alzheimer's disease, rheumatoid arthritis, nausea, cancer, seizure disorders, and cerebral ischemia (Zuardi; Amar, 3–15). Within the last five years, CBD research has escalated significantly, although federal regulations still prevent optimal access to the plant and its extracts. Some of the greatest strides have been made in CBD's use as a treatment for seizure disorders, neuropathic pain, cancer, and traumatic head injuries, although further clinical trials are still needed.

Success and Problems

Problems exist in that a specific cannabis strain, dosage method (inhalation, smoking, edibles, etc.), or dosing protocol cannot be established because of the unique way cannabis compounds work in different individuals. Despite this, general CBD:THC ratios have been established for different conditions and can be found online at Project CBD. This website also includes information on oil extracts and raw plant dosing.

Reasons for the individual responses to cannabis are described further in Chapter Three, but the one well-regarded explanation for varying effects is natural variation between individuals' endocannabinoid systems. While treatment success with CBD is making headlines, fine-tuning doses on an individual basis and working with different CBD:THC ratios for maximum results makes it difficult to predict outcomes. Speaking in a lecture series on cannabinoids in July 2014, Dr. Michelle Sexton explains that cannabinoids have potent antioxidant and anti-inflammatory properties. Cannabinoids also act as adaptogens that modulate the stress response, making their effects unique to the individual. Dr. Sexton describes CBD as having a sedating or calming effect, in contrast to the psychoactive effects of THC. She also emphasizes that no one dose of cannabinoids fits all and that there is not one specific strain, dose, or product type that works the same way for everyone (Lee and Sexton).

Restoring Homeostasis

Homeostasis refers to the body's amazing ability to establish and maintain a condition of balance or equilibrium within its internal environment, even when faced with external changes. In homeostasis, the body's various systems work together to maintain health. For example, skin cells, blood vessels, the thyroid gland, and other organs function synergistically to maintain an internal temperature of approximately 98.6 degrees Fahrenheit, regardless of the temperature outside.

One of the most often noted properties of CBD is its ability to restore and maintain homeostasis. It does this by correcting imbalances and mod-

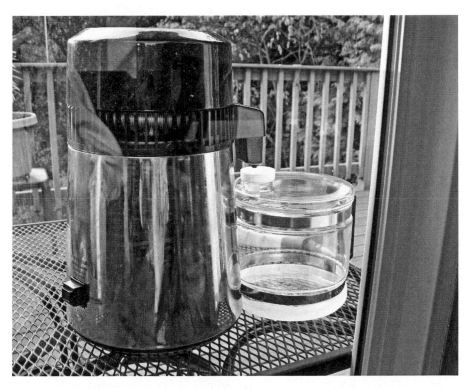

Distiller used to extract CBD oil (courtesy of Doug Flomer).

ulating nervous system and immune system functions. This fundamental property of CBD helps explain how the compound can benefit so many different diseases that seem unrelated. When disease is seen as a result of impaired homeostasis, it makes sense that CBD and other cannabinoids could have profound healing effects.

A Note on Seizure Disorders

In the majority of high–CBD strains currently used to treat seizure disorders (i.e., Charlotte's Web, ACDC), tremendous success has occurred in 15–20 percent of patients. Another 60–70 percent of treated patients have experienced a reduction in seizures, but not to the extent that would be considered a full success. Another 10 percent of patients have experienced no improvement (Lee, Martin, "The Cannabis Health Revolution"). More research is needed using various ratios of CBD to THC and possibly other cannabinoids and terpenes to confirm these findings. In addition, pediatric patients with seizure disorders need to be properly monitored by a physician for signs of improvement as well as any adverse effects. In the third session of The Cannabis Health Revolution course, Martin Lee emphasized that CBD used alone without THC can, in some instances, worsen seizures.

Several states have laws giving patients approval to use CBD alone, considering it safer because it lacks psychoactive properties. In a March 22, 2014, article on Project CBD, Martin Lee described problems with the CBD-only approach:

> Scientific research has established that CBD and THC interact synergistically and potentiate each other's therapeutic effects. And marijuana contains several hundred other compounds, including flavonoids, terpenes, and dozens of minor cannabinoids in addition to CBD and THC. Each of these compounds has particular healing attributes, but when combined they create what scientists refer to as an "entourage effect," so that the therapeutic impact of the whole plant exceeds the sum of its parts. Therein lies the basic fallacy of the CBD-only position.
>
> When we launched Project CBD four years ago, I thought the serendipitous rediscovery of CBD-rich cannabis would be the nail in the coffin of marijuana prohibition. I didn't anticipate that CBD-only laws would serve as a pretext to extend marijuana prohibition—under the guise, once again, of protecting the children [Lee, "The CBD Only Stampede," reprinted with permission].

Cannabidiol-Rich Strains

Under normal growing conditions, CBD is typically the second most prominent compound found in the cannabis plant. CBD's presence effectively reduces some of the psychoactive effects of THC and works together with THC and other cannabis phytochemicals to produce synergistic medical benefits. The concentration of CBD in cannabis extracts varies from trace quantities to amounts as high as 40 percent (Campos AC, Ferreira FR, and FS Guimarães, 1501; Grlic, 37). CBD used with even a small amount of THC is known to facilitate a return to homeostasis and thus natural healing. This ability is thought to derive primarily from CBD's modulating effects on the immune system, which are further described in Chapter Three.

Because little was known about CBD's health benefits until the discovery of the endocannabinoid system in the early 1990s, breeders have traditionally striven to grow cannabis plants with higher levels of THC and lower levels of CBD (Lee, "The Cannabis Health Revolution"). As a result, many of the current cannabis strains contain higher amounts of THC than baby boomers are used to, and breeders of medicinal cannabis are now seeking out high–CBD variants, with most strains coming from resin seeds harvested in Amsterdam (Frankel).

Today's consumers have a choice when it comes to buying medical marijuana. With the spotlight on CBD, many medical cannabis dispensaries carry products with higher CBD-to-THC ratios, typically around a 24:1 CBD:THC value. Such ratios are found in strains like Charlotte's Web, ACDC, and Avidekel in Israel. Although it has been demonstrated that CBD works best in conjunction with THC, consumers from all over the United States can buy products (see the Appendix) that contain only CBD; these products often still have benefits, though not to the extent of whole-plant extracts with THC. CBD oil and extracts made from industrial hemp are also more likely to contain contaminants.

Cannabis Plant Components

The main components derived from the *Cannabis sativa* L. plant include: fibrous stalk used for industrial fiber products; flowering buds and drug resin used for medicinal and psychoactive properties; and seed (including oil) used for fuel and food.

The commercial uses of hemp include textiles, foods, body lotions, plastics and building materials, paper, rope, and cordage. Hemp is a sustainable crop requiring no pesticides or herbicides. It contains only about 0.3–1.5 percent THC, which, combined with a relatively high CBD, content makes hemp completely unsuitable for psychoactive use. Different parts of the industrial hemp plant have varying uses. While the CBD in hemp can be extracted, the efficiency is far less than with true medicinal cannabis strains. In general, varieties of cannabis designated as industrial hemp are used for commercial purposes, whereas other cannabis strains are cultivated for medicinal or recreational use.

Hemp in America

Early American colonists introduced Indian hemp to North America. Similar to farmers in England, the early colonists were ordered by law to grow hemp for commercial purposes. By 1950, the cultivation of hemp came under federal control and was confined to Kentucky, Illinois, Minnesota, and Wisconsin (Goodman and Gilman, 2nd ed., 170–1). However, since the 1950s, hemp and marijuana have been categorized as identical, although in some cases efforts have been made to distinguish between the two.

Marijuana vs. Hemp

In the early 1950s, the most reliable test for marijuana in a substance was the ataxia test in dogs. The dog static ataxia test is historically significant. Studies using this model for identifying cannabis were among the first to suggest that THC produced behavioral effects by binding with a receptor, rather than by nonspecific membrane interactions. The administration of cannabinoid compounds to dogs causes them to weave back and forth while remaining in one place; the term "static ataxia" was coined to describe this peculiar collection of behaviors (Mackie, 2107–8).

Despite their clear differences, all cannabis plant products have traditionally fallen under the same restrictions. However, most of the world never stopped growing hemp, and today hemp for commercial use is primarily supplied by China, Hungary, England, Canada, Australia, France, Italy, Spain, Holland, Germany, Poland, Romania, Russia, Ukraine, India,

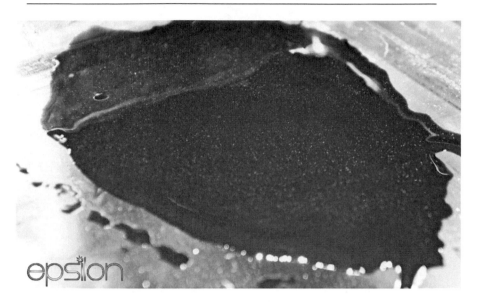

Essential oil extract of CBD-rich cannabis flower. The vibrant red appearance is often seen in clean, strong CBD-rich extracts (courtesy of Dave Mapes, Epsilon Apothecaries).

and other countries throughout Asia. In the United States, imported hemp products can be sold, but restrictions on growing the plant remain under strong government control.

Besides the interest in CBD:THC ratios, strains are being studied based on other cannabinoids and terpenes. It has long been known that different strains, chemical varieties, or cultivars of cannabis have different psychoactive and therapeutic effects, which can be explained both by individual responses and the composition of a particular strain's phytochemicals. For instance, some strains with high amounts of cannabigerol (CBG) are being studied for their use in prostate cancer (Russo, "Cannabis Strains").

The nonprofit Hemp Industries Association issued a statement in 2014 explaining the differences between hemp and cannabis to ensure that medical consumers buy the correct products. Their concern is that consumers often confuse hemp oil, a nutritious food product from seeds, with legal CBD oils from industrial hemp. This confusion arises because both are low in THC, are derived from hemp, and contain CBD (although seed oils have far less or even none compared to oils extracted from stalks, stems, or flowers specifically for CBD). Eric Steenstra, executive director of Hemp Industries Association, emphasized in a separate statement the necessity for consumers to understand the difference between CBD extracts and hemp oil. He requested that makers of CBD products brand and market their products truthfully and clearly, so as not to increase the confusion surrounding CBD products in the marketplace (Rucke).

Steenstra reported that although hemp oil does contain low levels of CBD, typically less than 25 parts per million (ppm), CBD extracts "are produced either directly from cannabis flowers that are up to 15 percent CBD (150,000 ppm), or indirectly as a co-product of the flowers and leaves that are mixed in with the stalks during hemp stalk processing for fiber" (Rucke).

Medicinal Cannabis CBD Oil vs. Industrial Hemp CBD Oil

CBD oil extracted from *Cannabis sativa*, which is available through medical dispensaries, is recommended over industrial hemp for medicinal use. Hemp extractions are legally sold online and thus are far more accessible to the general public. However, the most popular brands have been implicated in contamination problems, and the source of the hemp has also been called into question. In addition, CBD extracted from hemp seeds contains oxalic acid, which can be harmful to children with autism (Bluebird Botanicals). For this reason, manufacturers often dissolve CBD extracts in olive oil.

CBD-Rich Products, THCA, and CBDA

For medicinal uses, especially in seizure disorders and post–traumatic stress disorders, cannabis products with more CBD than THC are highly desirable. Specific strains such as Charlotte's Web and ACDC have ratios of CBD to THC of around 24:1, although extracts with lower CBD:THC ratios than those seen in Charlotte's Web are also used effectively for patients with seizure disorders. Strains containing more CBD than THC are called CBD-rich products, although the term high–CBD is also popular and both are used interchangeably in practice.

In its natural state, the living cells of fresh and dried cannabis contain the water-soluble form of THC, which is called THC carboxylic acid or

THC acid (THCA). It does not have psychoactive properties. If resin is present on the leaves, stems, or buds, the raw form of cannabis will have psychoactive properties.

THCA is a stable compound and breaks down into neutral THC very slowly. For decarboxylation (removing the carboxylic acid side chain from the molecule) to occur and turn THCA into its psychoactive form, cannabis must be heated to above 212 degrees Fahrenheit. As a neutral compound, THC is no longer soluble in water, although it is soluble in ethanol and fatty liquids (Clarke and Merlin 2013, 213).

Edible cannabis products intended to have a psychoactive effect must be mixed with a solvent or carrier (such as milk or other fats) to facilitate absorption. Eating the raw plant does not provide psychoactive properties because THCA is not decarboxylated efficiently through digestion. Thankfully, THCA and CBDA have their own unique medicinal benefits, including fighting cancer.

Cannabidiolic acid or CBD acid (CBDA) is a natural compound found in plants of the genus *Cannabis*. It is structurally similar to CBD, differing only by the addition of a carboxylic acid group added to the central ring. CBDA is produced by the oxidocyclization of cannabigerolic acid (CBGA) by CBDA synthase, a naturally occurring enzyme found in cannabis. CBDA is particularly effective in protocols used to treat multiple sclerosis and in seizure disorders.

The Dual Nature of Cannabis and CBD

Martin Lee describes the cannabis plant as a trickster with a dual nature that's not well understood (Lee and Sexton). For instance, Dr. Sexton states cannabis is an adaptogen, meaning it has bimodal or bidirectional effects, such as strengthening a weak immune system or balancing an overactive immune system. Another duality is that despite the plant's illegality, the legitimacy of cannabis as a medicinal herb is now established with its 2014 inclusion as a botanical medicine in the American Herbal Pharmacopoeia (AHP). The Cannabis Monograph in the AHP establishes a foundation and baseline for the ways in which health care professionals may utilize cannabis therapy and treatment in patients. Numerous studies and trials described in Chapter Eight also establish legitimacy.

As a trickster, cannabis can take on variable forms. Hemp and cannabis are essentially the same species but are non-identical twins. Plant constituents can also work for or against one another. As mentioned, CBD can either increase or decrease the effects of THC, depending on when the dose is given. Another example is the cannabinoid cannabidivarin (CBDV), a homolog of CBD, which has no psychoactive properties and blocks THC at receptors, inhibiting its effects. Some studies show that botanical cannabis extracts containing all of the plant's phytochemical compounds are more therapeutic. However, in a few cases, CBDA used alone exerts stronger therapeutic effects.

Dual properties of cannabis abound in the medical literature and include stimulant, depressant, sedative, antidepressant, analgesic, anti-rheumatic, diuretic, aphrodisiac, affection and pleasure inducer, anti-emetic, and anti-inflammatory.

Summary

Cannabidiol (CBD) is the second most abundant cannabinoid phytochemical found in the cannabis plant. Because it does not contain psychoactive properties, growers began to breed CBD out of cannabis strains in the 1970s. However, with new knowledge of its astonishing therapeutic potential, growers are producing varieties with a high CBD content for use in treating seizure disorders, cancer, rheumatism, post–traumatic stress disorders, neuropathic pain, head injuries, and other conditions. CBD works best used in conjunction with THC, and the recommended ratio of CBD to THC depends on the condition as well as the unique chemistry of the individual. Used as oil, CBD is best obtained from cannabis buds and leaves from CBD-rich cannabis plants rather than from industrial hemp, which contains smaller amounts of CBD and may contain impurities.

Two

Cannabis Botany, Taxonomy and Growth

Since its first medical description centuries ago, considerable disagreement has existed regarding the scientific classification of cannabis. Once grouped with the mulberry plant, cannabis has since found its rightful place in a family that also contains hops and nine other genera. Chapter Two focuses on the botany of cannabis, including its ancient origins, the most widely accepted classifications, the various cultivars or strains, plant growth and harvest, and the properties of the various plant parts.

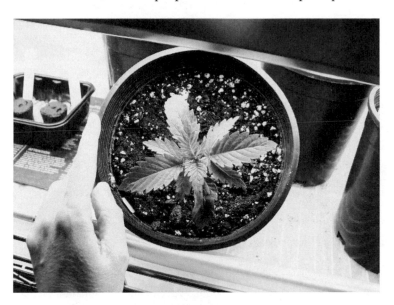

Early growth of *C. indica* (courtesy Doug Flomer).

The Cannabis Plant

Cannabis is one of the oldest cultivated economic plants, providing edible seed and fiber used for the production of rope, clothing, oil, soap, and paper. The flowering buds and leaves provide phytochemicals with medicinal and psychoactive properties. Despite restrictions mandated in the past 90 years making its cultivation and use largely illegal, cannabis has spread to every continent and most nations. It is regularly consumed by millions of people. In 2002, 48 percent of high school seniors in the United States reported some use of cannabis. This number is thought to be under-reported due to many high school students dropping out before 12th grade (O'Brien, 623).

Cannabis Classification

Cannabis is classified as belonging to the family Cannabaceae and the genus *Cannabis*. Although classification varies in different parts of the world, there is a general agreement that there are three species: *Cannabis sativa, Cannabis indica*, and *Cannabis ruderale* (Merlin and Clark, 312–5; Grinspoon and Bakalar, 1). The classifications are described in greater detail in the section on plant taxonomy later in this chapter. Cannabis strains are usually described as *C. indica, C. sativa*, or cannabis hybrids (which contain a mixture of types, usually a combination of *C.indica* and *C. sativa*).

The scientific classification of cannabis is still considered controversial. According to the *2014 American Herbal Pharmacopoeia for Cannabis Inflorescence,* cannabis has one highly variable species, *C. sativa*, with two subspecies, sativa and indica. In general, *C. indica* refers to plants with high levels of THC, while the name *C. sativa* has generally been applied to plants with a high yield of bast (phloem) fibers in the stem and a relatively high CBD-to-THC ratio (American Herbal Pharmacopoeia, 2).

Cannabis Terminology

The word cannabis is derived from the Greek word *kannabis*, which is related to the Sanskrit word *canna*, which means fragrant cane; *kannabosm* (Aramaic for fragrant cane) is referred to in the Old Testament as an ingredient of holy anointing oil (Lee, *Smoke*, 5). Common names for cannabis include the resin-rich *hashish* (an Arabic term for herb-eater) and *kief* for the plant resin; *charas* (WSJ Administrator), which is hand-made in Afghanistan, Pakistan, Nepal, and India from live resin-coated cannabis buds with very high concentrations of THC; *ganga bhang* for a cannabis-infused cordial; *ma* or *ma ta* as the name used in China by Shen Nung in 2000 BC; and *ghanga*, an Ayurvedic term for the plant resin mixed into a compound with clarified butter or ghee (Goodman and Gilman, 2nd ed., 170).

The term marijuana used in the United States refers to the psychoactive plant products and is said to be a corruption of the Portuguese word *mariguango*, meaning intoxicant (Goodman and Gilman, 2nd ed., 170). Since the 1950s, marijuana cigarettes have been called reefers, muggles, weed, tea, gage, sticks, and brownies (Goodman and Gilman, 2nd ed., 170).

In the 1930s, a man named Harry Anslinger, a former railroad police officer and prohibition agent, was appointed to head the new Bureau of Narcotics. He attempted to give marijuana a racist slant, associating it with Mexicans, gunfights, and loco weed, which is an entirely different plant, by using the term *marihuana* (Kuipers, 172; Gray). While it is still spelled incorrectly in some official documents, marijuana is the preferred spelling, and cannabis is the preferred term when referring to the cannabis plant.

The term "sinsemilla" is derived from the Spanish phrase meaning "without seed." Sinsemilla is the name most commonly used for seedless cannabis, which can be produced in female plants by separating them from males of the species.

Plant Components

Each cannabis plant consists of seven major plant sections. These include the flowers, stems, leaves, seeds, trichomes, roots, and main cola. The plant cola (bud site or terminal bud) is the part of a female cannabis plant where the flowers or buds grow together tightly on a single branch. In plant physiology, this is known as the terminal bud. Strong, healthy plants commonly form one main cola, arising from the center of the branching structure, with smaller colas forming around the outside of the plant. Various trimming techniques can be used to increase the number

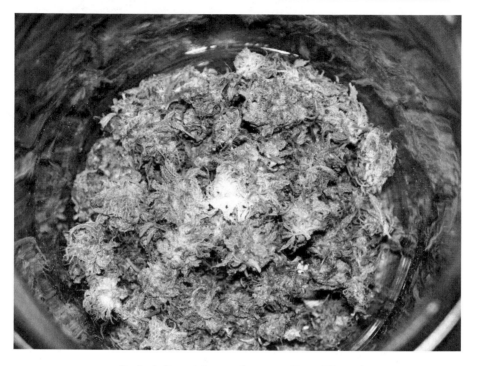

Resin-laden trichomes (courtesy Doug Flomer).

of large colas that endow a plant. Female plants also have a pistil and calyx, which are involved in pollination. The chemical constituents (cannabinoids, terpenes, amino acids, etc.) of cannabis are described in Chapter Five.

CANNABIS INFLORESCENCE

Cannabis inflorescence, which is commonly called bud, refers to the fixed pattern in which clusters of flowers are arranged on a stem. Depending on the genetics of the particular plant and its environmental conditions, the plant presents with a variable density and size of bracts (flower shoots) interspersed in the inflorescence.

TRICHOMES AND HARVESTING

Resinous, glandular oil glands called trichomes occur in maturing female, hermaphrodite, and some male plants. Non-glandular trichomes primarily occur in males and cover the staminate calyx. Trichomes can be described as hair-like projections, which act as an evolutionary sticky shield, protecting the plant and its seeds from the dangers of the environment, such as insects, and allowing cannabis to reproduce. The chemicals in glandular trichomes are unpalatable and prevent animals from eating the plants. These chemicals also act as a natural fungicide. Cannabinoid production begins in the trichomes, and the cannabinoids are later released to various plant parts (Clarke, 136).

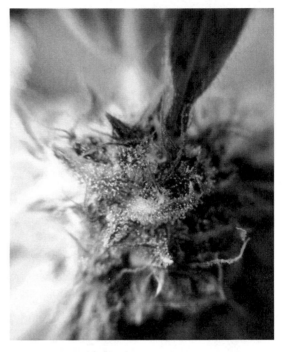

Cannabis trichomes on Pit Bull, a *C. Indica* strain (courtesy Doug Flomer).

Trichomes physically appear as crystalline droplets that hug the plant surface. They first emerge on small leaves and stems. As the flowering phase continues over several weeks, oil glands develop on the more mature parts of the plant, including the outer portion of the bracts, the smaller leaves, and the first calyxes. The trichomes that develop on calyxes appear as stalks with bulbous caps. At this time, more and more trichome-covered calyxes develop and create densely packed clusters, called "bud." As cannabis plants enter the final stages of their life cycle, the calyxes begin to swell and ripen, while more and more resin glands continue to develop on the surface. The window of peak maturity in cannabis and the best time for harvesting is when trichome development and the level of THC (and/or CBD) production have reached their maximum points. Resin-laden trichomes can be separated from the plant at harvest and used to make hashish and hash oil.

Hemp and Cannabis

Hemp describes the fibrous plant stalk or stem, which has no psychoactive properties and is used to produce edible seeds and sturdy fibers for cordage, rope, and clothing. Hemp seed can be processed into protein- and fatty acid-rich food for humans and animals. Oil from the seeds is used for fuel, lotions, lacquers, varnishes, and soap.

Known for their own healing properties, hemp seeds contain an abundance of omega–3 essential fatty acids, correcting the modern dietary imbalance that results in too high a ratio of omega–6 to omega–3 fatty acids. Linoleic acid is the primary omega–6 fatty acid that occurs in hemp seed. Gamma linolenic acid (GLA) is also found in smaller amounts. These fatty acids have potent anti-inflammatory properties. In addition, hemp seeds contain arginine, which protects against endothelial dysfunction and cardiovascular disease. Hemp seed is recommended for improving cardiac health, reducing inflammation, and reducing symptoms of eczema (Gamonski, 93–94).

Plants grown for industrial hemp and plants grown for cannabis extracts and bud have different growth requirements. Cannabis plants intended for recreational or medical use must be grown in generally warm and humid environments in order to produce the desired quantity and quality of flowering buds. Since industrial hemp does not contain these buds, and the hardy parts of the hemp plant are desired, the hemp plant can be grown in a wider range of areas. Industrial hemp grows best on fields that provide high yields for corn crops, which includes most of the Southwest, Southeast, and Northeast United States. Often, farmers rotate the two crops. In addition, since industrial hemp can use male plants as well as female plants, these crops produce a higher yield. Growers often remove male plants to prevent pollination and produce resin-laden sinsemilla crops for medicinal cannabis.

HEMP PRODUCTION

For the average farmer in the 1800s, industrial hemp was difficult to process. In 1800s England, many farmers preferred paying a fine to having to grow hemp. In the United States, plantation owners occasionally paid wages to slaves to encourage hemp production (Lee, *Smoke* 19). When Thomas Jefferson retired to Virginia after two terms as president in 1809 and attempted to raise hemp, he quickly had to abandon the project, finding it too labor-intensive even with the help of slaves (Lee, *Smoke*, 19).

Despite the processing obstacles, by 1850 hemp was America's third-largest crop, exceeded only by cotton and tobacco. However, by the time the Civil War began in 1861, cotton had wended its way into the textile marker and was soon joined by flax. Consequently, by the late 19th century, fiber hemp had begun to decline in commercial value. Around this time, with non-fiber cannabis plants' greater availability, its reputation as a medical tonic began to rise.

Plant Origins

In their book *Cannabis, Evolution and Ethnobotany*, Clarke and Merlin use botanical, ecological, and archeological evidence to hypothesize that cannabis originated in one of the more temperate and well-watered areas of ancient Central Asia.

In 2008, a team of international researchers reported finding approximately two pounds of well-preserved flower tops, shoots, and leaves of cannabis buried about 27 centuries ago alongside a light-haired, blue-eyed Caucasian man (likely a Gushi shaman) in a remote graveside in the Yanghai Tombs near Turpan, Xinjiang-Uighur Autonomous Region, China (Jiang et al., 414–6; Russo et al., 4171–4; Lee, *Smoke*, 4).

Greg Green describes an earlier existence of cannabis. Hunting nets used by the Gravettians, an ancient culture of the European Upper Paleolithic (old Stone Age), date back to 24,980 to 22,870 BC (Green, 2). Green hypothesizes that cannabis grew wild, originating in the Himalayas. After its introduction to China, the first domesticated cannabis strains were bred 6500 years ago in Mongolia (Green, 2–3).

H. L. Li describes the center of domestication as probably Pan-p'-o, China, in 4500 BC (Li, "Origin and Use," 293). As a cultivated plant, cannabis had a variety of uses. Aside from its application as a fiber and medicine, cannabis was considered one of the major "grains of the ancients" and was eaten in the form of gruel (Li, "An archaeological," 438).

MEDICINAL ORIGINS

The first written reference to the medicinal use of cannabis dates back to the year 2737 BC. In this early report, Emperor Shen Nung recorded medical uses of cannabis in his pharmacopoeia, *Pen Ts'ao Ching*. Shen Nung called cannabis (*ma*) one of the "Supreme Elixirs of Immortality" and recommended its use for female weakness, gout, rheumatism, malaria, constipation, spasms, beri-beri, and absentmindedness. He also cautioned that, taken in excess, psychoactive cannabis resin (Clarke and Merlin, 6) could make people "see demons" (Lee, *Smoke*, 5).

Cannabis Growth

Considered an annual herbaceous plant propagated from seed, cannabis grows from medium to tall height (approximately three to twenty feet) in both temperate and tropical climates, particularly in open sunny environments with well-drained soil, essential nutrients, and water. Growth is variable because environmental influences strongly affect how individual cannabis plants develop. For instance, in substandard soil, mature plants capable of producing seed may only grow to eight inches (Clarke and Merlin, 13).

The growing season of cannabis typically lasts four to six months and results in plants reaching heights of about 20 feet, depending on the subspecies and gender. Wild or feral cannabis strains often exist near human populations in agricultural lands, exposed riverbanks, roadsides, and in sunny meadows.

Cannabis seeds typically are planted in the spring and germinate in three to seven days. Seedlings emerge from the ground by the straightening of the hypocotyl or embryonic stem. The cotyledons or seed leaves are unequal in size, narrowed to base and rounded or blunt at the tip (Clarke, 1981, 1). About one-half to three inches above the seed leaflet, the first true leaves arise as a pair of single leaflets facing in opposite directions, each with their own stem or petiole. Within two to three months following germination, cannabis plants show a vigorous growth response to increased day length, which is characterized by an increasing number of leaflets on each plant leaf.

As the season progresses with shorter periods of daylight (12 to 14 hours or less with longer nights of 10 to 12 hours), the plants begin to flower in response to critical daylight periods that vary among different strains. Flowering marks completion of the cannabis life cycle (Clarke and Watson, 5). From there the process of deriving the plant products begins. See the section on plant gender later in this chapter to learn how plant products are derived. For readers desiring more information on cannabis growth, in his 2010 book *The Cannabis Grow Bible*, Greg Green comprehensively describes each step and requirement of cannabis growth.

The optimal harvest time depends on the types and amounts of desired phytochemicals and the environmental conditions of the crop (American Herbal Pharmacopoeia, 28). Growers at the government's University of Mississippi cannabis farm analyze their raw material daily to determine the optimal time of harvest for peak THC acid (THCA) concentrations. In general, optimal harvest time occurs when the plant buds reach full maturity. At this time at least 75 percent of the stigmas should have turned browned and shriveled (American Herbal Pharmacopoeia, 28).

Cannabis Seeds

The fruit or seed of cannabis is partially encased by the bract. The calyx is reduced to a seed coat variously patterned in gray, brown, or black. Seeds typically measure $\frac{1}{12}$ to $\frac{1}{4}$ inches in length and $\frac{1}{24}$ to $\frac{1}{6}$ inches in width. Their weights vary from 600 seeds/gram in wild strains to 15 seeds/gram in cultivated varieties. Larger seeds have long been used to produce edible grains (Clarke and Merlin, 16).

Landrace Cannabis Strains

The term "landrace" refers to genetic integrity, characterized by recognizable morphology. Unique landraces differ in their adaptation to soil type, seed germination, date of maturity, height, nutritive value, use, and other properties, including genetic diversity (Green, 3).

Historical documents from around the world indicate that cannabis has lived alongside humans for thousands of years, cultivated for religious and medicinal purposes. Many growers believe that the earliest cannabis strains sprouted in Central Asia as well as the Hindu Kush regions of Afghanistan and Pakistan and eventually spread to other areas, including South America, Asia, Jamaica, Africa, and even Russia. These indigenous strains are known as landraces, in contrast to feral strains.

A landrace strain refers to a local variety of cannabis that has adapted to the environment of its geographic location, such as the Kush strains of

Afghanistan. This accounts for genetic variation between landrace strains, which have been crossbred to produce the cannabis varieties seen today. Landrace strains are often named after their native region, such as Afghani and Thai. Centuries after reports of their early use, traces of these forefather strains are sometimes detectable and found in the names of their crossbred descendants. A combination of environmental conditions and selective breeding by native populations gave rise to these stable varieties, the forefathers of all modern strains. Until its prohibition, cannabis remained a cultural cornerstone in these areas of the world.

Today's cannabis market rarely encounters pure landrace strains, although modern cultivars, such as Kush, Master Kush, and Hash Plant, can evolve into landrace strains when seed harvested from the same crop cultivar is used over time (Green, 4). The reasons pure landrace strains are rarely seen today include (1) hybridization, which strips the plant of its natural genetic profile and (2) indoor growing, which often subjects the plants to conditions that alter growth and the development of its natural phytochemicals.

During the 1970s and 80s, growers worldwide began collecting landrace strains to breed in their own local gardens. These strains, called heirlooms, were then propagated in other environments like Hawaii and California. Landrace strains include:

Table 2.1
Cannabis Landrace Strains

Hindu Kush	variety of *Cannabis indica*
Pua or Pure Afghan	variety of *Cannabis indica*
Lamb's Bread	variety of *Cannabis sativa* that originated in Jamaica
Acapulco Gold	hybrid variety from Mexico
Durban Poison and Malawi	varieties of *Cannabis sativa* from Africa
Panama Red	variety of *Cannabis sativa* from Central America.

The Ethnobotany of Cannabis

Ethnobotany refers to the ways in which civilizations interact with plants. Cannabis was one of the first crops grown in Eurasia. Ancient cannabis fiber discovered in China is typically found as scraps of cordage, cloth, or paper. In addition, cannabis seeds were used as both food and oil, and the flowering plant and leaves were used as medicine. In Korea, cannabis fiber (*sambae; da ma*) has been used for thousands of years to make textiles. Ancient cannabis fibers have been unearthed as far west as Turkey. Artifacts dating back to the time of the Phrygians, an Aryan tribe who invaded Turkey around 1000 BC contain hemp fiber (Abel, 23).

Euphoric Properties

Paleolithic populations in Central Asia first discovered the euphoriant properties of cannabis. This discovery may have happened while they tasted resin as they gathered seed or prepared it for use as food. Fresh and dried cannabis has little psychoactive potency because it contains the acid forms of the plant's cannabis constituents. For cannabis to become psychoactive, it must be heated to temperatures above 212 degrees Fahrenheit. Burning cannabis or heating it for long periods of low-temperature cooking can convert water-soluble inactive acid THC (THCA) into its neutral psychoactive form (THC).

Plant Taxonomy

The first botanical illustration of cannabis in Western literature appears as a drawing found in a Byzantine manuscript from AD 512 written by Dioscorides, whose *Materia Medica* is the foundation for all modern pharmacopeias (Lee, *Smoke*, 5). The botanist Carl Lannaeus christened the plant *Cannabis sativa* in 1753.

The cannabis plant is assigned as the type genus in the small family Cannabaceae. This family consists of only two genera: *Cannabis* and the hops plant, *Humulus* (Clarke and Merlin, 312). As the type genus, cannabis defines the characteristics of its family.

Cannabis includes a group of flowering herbs that vary in their morphology and physiology. Cannabaceae was formerly included in the fig and nettle families, but has since been recognized as a distinct family. Recent research suggested reclassifying cannabis into the Celtidaceae family, but differences in their growth form precluded this (Clarke and Merlin, 312). The production of THC in cannabis, which is responsible for the plant's psychoactive properties, is thought to have arisen from a single mutation, creating the psychoactive-inducing B_T allele (Clarke and Merlin, 331).

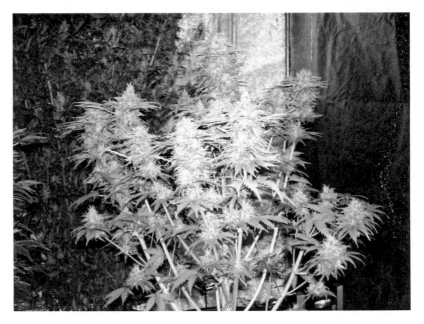

Healthy cannabis plant near harvest (courtesy Doug Flomer).

The accepted species of the genus *Cannabis* include *Cannabis sativa* L. (the L indicating this Latin species name was provided by the Swiss taxonomist Carolus Linnaeus in 1753); *Cannabis indica*; and *Cannabis ruderalis*. In 1785, Lamarck described *Cannabis sativa* as a taller, more fibrous plant, whereas *Cannabis indica* was depicted as a shorter plant with broad leaves and more psychoactivity. In 1924, Janischevsky first described *Cannabis ruderalis* as a very small weedy variety that was not cultivated. He reported that it produced oils in glands near the base of each seed. *C. ruderalis* is thought to have been hybridized with other feral strains (Clarke and Merlin, 316). All of the cannabis species and their subspecies are capable of producing THC and CBD, with *C. indica* producing the highest amounts of these phytochemicals.

Cannabis plants include Narrow leaf drug (NLD), Broad leaf drug (BLD), and Broad leaf hemp (BLH) varieties. These are thought to have evolved from a common prototype drug gene pool derived from the putative drug ancestor or PDA. (Clarke and Merlin, 321). From an evolutionary viewpoint, the hemp varieties have much less THC and more CBD content, whereas the drug types have far more THC than CBD. Therefore, the varieties are commonly known as "dope vs. rope" strains.

Plant Gender

Normally, cannabis is a dioecious plant, which means that male (staminate) and female (pistillate) flowers develop on separate plants. Occasionally, as a result of genetics, hermaphrodite plants containing both sex characteristics emerge. Plants containing both male and female characteristics can also develop from nutrient deficiencies or excesses, as well as unusual climate changes. These stressful events often trigger hermaphrodite characteristics or other problems in cannabis plants.

Gender is typically not determined until the cannabis plants begin to flower, although sophisticated analytical techniques (such as DNA profiling) and some growth hints can help determine gender earlier. The first sign of flowering is characterized by the appearance of undifferentiated flower primordia that emerge along the main stem at the nodes or intersections of the petiole, behind the leaf spur or stipule. Primordia in female plants often appear two weeks earlier than seen in male plants.

As they mature, the undifferentiated primordia soon change into staminate primordia (male plants); undifferentiated vegetative growth; and pistillate primordia (females). The male plants at this time develop a curved, claw shape, followed by the appearance of round, pointed flower buds having five radial segments. The females show enlargement of a symmetrical tubular calyx or floral sheath. These early calyxes tend to lack paired pistils for catching pollen, but with maturity, the paired pistils appear. The female plants are typically shorter with more branches than the male. Female plants are leafy at the top, with many leaves surrounding the flowers. Male plants have fewer leaves near the top, with few, if any, leaves along the flowering limbs (Clarke, 6).

Typically, cannabis crops contain equal amounts of male and female plants (Clarke, 8). However, under conditions of extreme stress (nutrient excess or deficiency, climate changes), mutilation, and altered light cycles, this gender ratio can change. As mentioned, such stressors can also result in more plants with both male and female components.

MALE VS. FEMALE PLANTS

The female flowers appear as two long white, yellow, or pink pistils, which protrude from the fold of a membranous calyx. The calyx is covered with resin exuding glandular trichomes (hairs). Pistillate flowers emerge in pairs, one on each side of the petiole behind the bracts (reduced leaves), which help conceal the flowers.

Male flowers, which emerge up to a month before female flowers, have five small petals of yellow, white or green that hang down and make up the calyx. The exterior surface of the staminate calyx is covered with non-glandular trichomes. The pollen grains are nearly spherical, small, and slightly yellow. Soon after shedding its pollen, the male plant, which can also produce resin, dies, while the female may mature up to five months after viable flowers are formed if little or no fertilization occurs (Clarke, 7).

Pollination

Just prior to pollination, the pollen nucleus divides to produce a small reproductive cell and a large vegetative cell, both of which can be found in pollen grain. Germination occurs 15 to 20 minutes after contact with a pistil. At this time the reproductive cell enters the pollen tube and migrates towards the ovule. The generative cell divides into two gametes as it travels through the pollen tube.

Pollination of the female flower is responsible for the browning, shriveling, and eventual loss of the male plant's paired stigmas and also a swelling of the tubular tract inside which the fertilized ovule is enlarging in females. After about three to six weeks, the seed matures. Growers can then harvest the seeds or wait until the seeds drop to the ground. Seeds are usually viable for three to five years of storage at room temperature, ten years when refrigerated, and for decades with uninterrupted freezing (Clarke and Merlin, 16).

Unfertilized female plants, whether through separation from males or through an accident of nature, are known as sinsemilla. As the unfertilized calyxes swell, the glandular trichomes on the surface grow and secrete aromatic resin, which has a high THC content. The mature, pungent, sticky floral clusters are harvested, dried, and put into use (Clarke, 10).

Although female plants have been long been prized for their abundant resin (and higher THC yield), male plants can also produce plants rich in cannabinoids. Stoney Girl Gardens reports that their Blue Bull males tested at 11 percent CBD and up to 6 percent THC (Valley). They plan to continue growing males for oil production because they turn over so much faster than females and possess the sought-after high CBD:THC ratio.

34

Plant Products

Lacking appreciable amounts of THC, hemp has been widely used in housing construction. Both the long bast fibers and woody inner core have unique uses. Silica leached from the soil by the cannabis plant combined with unslaked lime forms a chemical bond and a fireproof, waterproof product with properties similar to those of cement. Hemp is also used to produce textiles, fiber, rope, cordage, paper (from tissue paper to cardboard), protein-rich food, and clean-burning ethanol fuel (Earleywine, 127).

Cannabis buds and leaves can be processed into a number of different forms, including marijuana, hashish, and hash oil, as well as cannabis extracts, oils, and tinctures. Residents of India distinguish products based on what plant part they are made from. *Bhang* refers to the dried leaves of the plant, comparable to marijuana in America. *Ganja* refers to the resin-laden tops of female plants in India, although in Jamaica, this term applies to the leaves. *Charas* refers to the dried resin (hashish) separated from the flowers and pressed together. Hash oil is produced by boiling hashish or buds in a solvent and straining the contents through a filter. The solvent is then allowed to evaporate (Earleywine, 127). Hash oil, while concentrated and rich in THC, requires glass pipes for smoking and often retains traces of flammable solvents like butane, making its use potentially unsafe and unhealthy.

Plant Phytochemicals

Cannabis contains more than 1,000 natural compounds, including 120 aromatic terpenes, and more than 100 cannabinoids. Several subclasses of cannabinoids have been identified, the most prominent being the delta–9-tetrahydrocannabinol (THC) type, with nine cannabinoids in this group. The second most prominent group is the cannabidiol (CBD) type, which contains seven cannabinoids. The acid precursors and cannabinoid homologues have also been identified (ElSohly, 29). See Chapter Five for more information on cannabis phytochemicals and their properties.

In ancient times, medicinal benefits, such as relief of migraine and rheumatic pain, were attributed to the entire plant or its drug resin. Beginning in the 1960s, when scientists began to isolate the individual plant components and identify their structure, specific effects were assigned to the various cannabinoids. In some disorders, including seizure disorders and cancer, both CBD and THC are used and show beneficial effects. The task of scientists now is to determine what CBD:THC ratios work best for different conditions and what administration forms are optimal. Terpenes and other cannabis phytochemicals are also being investigated for their medicinal properties.

A great deal of medicinal cannabis research has been accomplished in the last decade, and it has become apparent that cannabis as a form of herbal medicine is here to stay. Still, Lester Grinspoon, MD, cautions that hemp oil products sold online solely on the basis of anecdotal evidence can be harmful and lack efficacy (Grinspoon, "Medical Marijuana"). In particular, oil containing less than 0.3 percent THC with high amounts of CBD can be legally be sold in the United States and is widely available through online sources. Cannabis products derived from specific strains that have been studied in clinical trials are recommended and should be obtained from medical dispensaries or clinics. They should also be consumed with the guidance of a naturopathic or integrationist physician who has experience with their use.

Summary

Cannabis, along with hops, belongs to the family Cannabaceae. The three recognized species of the genus *Cannabis* include *Cannabis sativa*, *Cannabis indica*, and *Cannabis ruderalis*. Plants from all of these species contain variable amounts of plant phytochemicals. Cannabis originated in Central Asia centuries ago. Early on, hemp was used to make textiles. The seed was used to produce oils for fuel, and the plant's leaves and flowering buds were used for their psychoactive and medicinal effects. Cannabis grows well in temperate climates, but plants grown for industrial hemp can tolerate harsher conditions.

While the uses of cannabis remain the same as they did centuries ago, there is a renewed interest in and exploration of the medicinal benefits of the cannabis plant's phytochemicals and the use of hemp as a sustainable crop for fuels and textiles. Specific cannabis strains are being bred and investigated in medical studies. The goal is to provide products that can be used under the guidance of a qualified physician for a wide range of medical conditions.

THREE

The Endocannabinoid Receptor System

A network of systems, including the cardiovascular system, the immune system, the endocrine system, and the nervous system, control the many diverse functions of the human body. Cells that make up a particular system communicate with neurotransmitters, hormones, other cells, and drugs to carry out specific effects within the system and other systems as well. For example, both psychological and physical stress affect the nervous system, which in turn modulates the immune system as well as a recently discovered chemical messaging network called the endocannabinoid system (ECS).

Both phytocannabinoids (derived from the cannabis plant) and endocannabinoids (cannabinoids produced within the body) communicate through this system to produce specific physiological effects. Chapter Three describes the key components of the endocannabinoid system and explains how specific phytochemicals in cannabis, such as delta–9-tetrahydrocannabinol (THC) and cannabidiol (CBD), are able to evoke their intended physiological effects.

The Endocannabinoid System (ECS)

Although the first hints of the ECS did not emerge until 1988 with the discovery of the cannabinoid receptor, the endocannabinoid system is an ancient neuronal signaling system in which cells of the nervous system communicate with each other and also their environment. This system, which works to maintain homeostasis (a stable internal environment that promotes balanced health), developed over millions of years ago in humans and other mammals and dates back to our first ancestors.

The ECS influences general health and plays important functions in neurodegenerative and neuroinflammatory disorders, such as Alzheimer's disease, Parkinson's disease, amyotrophic lateral sclerosis (ALS), multiple sclerosis (MS), glaucoma, osteoporosis, seizure disorders, and cancer (Maccarone et al., 1380–1). It also modulates the immune system's cells, thereby offering protection against cancer and autoimmune diseases and reducing associated inflammation. Before the discovery of the ECS, cannabis research was limited. The idea that the phytochemicals in cannabis reacted with lipids in the cell membrane had been proposed by scientists but not supported by research until cannabinoid receptors were discovered. With the discovery of the ECS, the effects of cannabis were no longer shrouded in mystery. Thus, in recent years, the ECS has emerged as a key target of pharmacotherapy.

Cell Receptors and Drugs

For many years, researchers studied the effects of drugs without knowing for certain how their effects came to be. Parameters could be measured, such as a reduction in inflammation after an anti-inflammatory drug such as aspirin was given, but the mechanics behind these beneficial effects remained a mystery. The idea of receptors was proposed but not proven. For instance, in the early years of the 20th century, researchers hypothesized that the catecholamine compounds epinephrine and norepinephrine might be binding to receptor-like structures on cells to cause their well-documented effects on heart muscle.

As researchers later discovered, many drugs do bind to receptors. Receptors are proteins found on the cell surface or nucleus that act much like locks. When specific chemical compounds known as ligands (both endogenous, which are produced within the body, or exogenous, which are ingested from outside the body) bind to specific receptors, they open the lock, activating the receptor and eliciting a specific physiological action. Receptors allow cells to communicate with one another and with the environment. For any drug or chemical for which a receptor exists on human cells, upon its discovery, researchers want to know the reasons for its presence.

RECEPTOR-SPECIFIC ACTIONS

In 1948, Raymond Ahlquist discovered that there were two distinct receptors for catecholamine drugs that caused different responses in heart muscle. These receptors were named alpha- and beta-adrenergic receptors. Soon, drugs that could stimulate receptor activation (agonists) or block receptor activation (antagonists) were developed. One important example is the beta-adrenergic receptor antagonists (beta blockers) used to treat hypertension. These findings form the cornerstone of modern-day research into drug development. Researchers, on discovering a new cellular protein receptor, surmise that the body must also be producing an endogenous chemical that binds or reacts with this novel receptor.

THE OPIATE RECEPTOR

With the 1972 discovery of the opiate receptor by the pharmacologist Candace Pert at Johns Hopkins University, the effects of drugs on brain chemistry were further elucidated. Pert discovered how the body's endorphins as well as opiate drugs are able to bind to one or more of the opiate receptor subtypes on brain cells to alleviate pain and render feelings of bliss. This discovery led to a crucial understanding of how drugs interacted with structures within the brain.

DISCOVERY OF THE CANNABINOID RECEPTOR

In 1988, Allyn Howlett and William Devane from St. Louis University used radioimmunoassay techniques to characterize the existence of a cannabinoid receptor in a rat brain (Pacher, Batkai, and Kunos, 389–392; Lee, *Smoke*, 209). In 1990, Miles Herkenham and his team at the National Institute of Mental Health (NIMH) mapped the locations of a cannabinoid receptor system in several mammalian species, including man (Herkenham et al., 1932–4).

With these breakthrough findings, the hunt was on to find an endogenous chemical compound that acted as a ligand for the cannabinoid receptor. Typically, such compounds are found in the same area of the body in which the particular receptor was discovered. In 1990, researchers found that cannabinoid receptors are heterogeneously located throughout the brain and most dense in the forebrain areas associated with higher cognitive functions and in hindbrain areas associated with the control of motor and sensory functions of the autonomic nervous system.

The highest densities of cannabinoid receptor binding in the hindbrain were localized in the molecular layer of the cerebellar cortex and the dorsal motor nucleus of the vagus. The spinal cord showed very low levels of receptor binding. These findings indicate roles for cannabinoids in cognition and movement. Cannabinoid receptors are sparse in the lower brain-stem areas controlling heart and lung function. For this reason, cannabinoids used in excess cannot cause the respiratory depression and heart failure associated with other drug classes.

Structure of the Cannabinoid Receptor

Cannabinoid receptors belong to a class of cell membrane receptors called the G-Coupled Receptor Superfamily. Forty percent of all drugs react by binding to G protein-coupled receptors (Lee and Marcu). Similar to other such receptors, the cannabinoid receptors contain seven transmembrane-spanning domains.

Cannabinoid receptors are activated by three major groups of ligands (proteins that bind to receptors). These are endocannabinoids produced by our bodies; cannabis plant-derived cannabinoids such as THC and CBD; and synthetic cannabinoids such as HU-210 and JWH-133. These ligands can bind completely or partially to CB1 and CB2 receptors. Some ligands, especially synthetic ones, are selective for only one type of receptor. For example, JWH-133 is a selective CB2 agonist, whereas the phytocannabinoid THC activates both CB1 and CB2 receptors.

CANNABINOID RECEPTOR AGONISTS
AND ANTAGONISTS

Compounds that bind with and activate a cannabinoid receptor are called cannabinoid receptor agonists. Receptor antagonists are ligands (including drugs) that block or dampen agonist-mediated responses at the receptor, inhibiting the normal biological response that occurs when agonists bind to the receptor. Antagonists of the CB1 receptor were once researched for their anti-obesity effects (Pacher, Batkai, and Kunos, 401–6). A CB1 antagonist drug known as Rimonabant was briefly available in Europe for treating obesity, but problems with severe depression and suicidal thoughts in patients led to its quick withdrawal.

Endocannabinoid System Components

The endocannabinoid system is composed of various G protein-coupled transmembrane receptors; endogenous (produced naturally within the body) cannabinoids; transient receptor potential channels; melatonin and serotonin receptors; the PPARs (peroxisome proliferator-activated receptors); several orphan G protein-coupled receptors; and enzymes that catalyze the synthesis and breakdown of the system's components. Enzymes in this system include fatty acid amide hydrolase (FAAH); calcium-dependent trans-acylase; N-acyl-phosphatidylethanolamine phospholipase D (NaPE-PLD); and Pi-selective phospholipase C (Pi-PPL). One of the ways CBD influences health is by inhibiting the activity of FAAH, the enzyme that degrades anandamide. In this way, CBD increases natural anandamide levels and indirectly stimulates the classical cannabinoid receptors.

What's the Endocannabinoid System For?

The ECS's basic function is to direct us to eat, sleep, relax, forget, and protect, which are all functions needed for optimal health (Lee and Marcu). Considered a master regulator, the ECS regulates immune function, restores and maintains homeostasis, protects the brain and nervous system, modulates the transmission of neurotransmitters, and buffers the affects of stress (Lee, Martin, *The Cannabis Health Revolution*).

Endogenous Cannabinoids (Endocannabinoids)

The search for the elusive chemical compound (endogenous cannabinoid) has led to the discovery of several endogenous compounds or eicosanoids that bind selectively to cannabinoid receptors. The best studied of the endocannabinoids are:

1. N-Arachidonoylethanolamine (AEA; anandamide [from the Sanskrit word meaning bliss]) is a modified form of arachidonic acid with central nervous system actions similar to those of THC. It has great affinity for the CB1 receptor, where it serves as a partial agonist, and little affinity for the CB2 receptor.

2. 2-Arachidonoyl glycerol (2-AG) has peripheral actions similar to those of THC but, unlike anandamide, binds equally well to both CB1 and CB2 receptors.

Anandamide and 2-AG appear to function as neurotransmitters or neuromodulators, with an additional role of serving as retrograde synaptic messengers.

Other proposed endocannabinoids under investigation include: palmitoyl-ethanolamide, which appears to taper allergic reactions; docosatetraenylethanolamide; 2-arachidonylglyceryl ether (noladin ether); homo-gamma-linoenylethanolamide; and oleamide.

Endocannabinoids are derived from phospholipid precursors in cell membranes and are synthesized on demand rather than stored in the body. Evidence shows that tissue concentrations of endocannabinoids, cannabinoid receptor density, and/or cannabinoid receptor coupling efficiency increase in a range of disorders, including multiple sclerosis, certain types of pain, cancer, schizophrenia, post–traumatic stress disorders, some intestinal and cardiovascular diseases, excitotoxicity, and traumatic head injury ("Cannabis Pharmacology," S174).

Endocannabinoid Metabolism

Following the discovery of anandamide, researchers found that mammalian tissues contain a number of other fatty acid derivatives that behave as endogenous cannabinoids. Once endocannabinoids are released into the circulation and target cannabinoid receptors, they are removed from their site of action within the cells through a process of metabolism, which is facilitated by the endocannabinoid receptor system enzymes fatty acid amide hydrolase and monoacylglycerol lipase (Pertwee, "Cannabis Pharmacology," S168).

Most of the identified endocannabinoids activate cannabinoid receptors with the exception of virodhamine, which blocks them. Anandamide is also reported to activate the vanilloid TRPV1 receptor (Pertwee, "Cannabis Pharmacology," S169). Other synthetic compounds such as the Bayer molecule, BAY 38–7271, which activate both CB1 and CB2 receptors, have also been developed and are being investigated for their therapeutic benefits. For instance, the drug Sativex, a cannabis-based medicine that contains both delta–9-THC and CBD is licensed in Canada as adjunctive treatment for the symptomatic relief of neuropathic pain in adults with multiple sclerosis.

Cannabinoid Receptor Subtypes

Two types of cannabinoid receptor have been discovered. They are distinguished by differences in their predicted amino acid sequence, signaling mechanisms, distribution within the body's tissues, and their sensitivity to certain receptor agonists and antagonists (Howlett et al., 162).
Cannabinoid receptors include:

1. CB1 receptors, primarily found on cells of the central nervous system (CNS), which includes the brain and spinal cord. They are also found on cells in the liver, lungs, kidneys, adipose tissue, skeletal muscle, and reproductive organs of both males and females. CB1 receptors do not appear in the medulla oblongata, the part of the brain stem responsible for respiratory and cardiovascular functions. For this reason, there is no risk of respiratory or cardiovascular failure. CB1 receptors are considered the cause of the euphoric and anticonvulsive effects of cannabis. CB1 receptors are highly expressed on axons and axon terminals, positions that allow them to modulate neurotransmission. Endocannabinoids produced by neurons or glial cells mediate several forms of transient and persistent synaptic plasticity (ability of synaptic connections to increase). CB1 receptors have also been found on immune system cells (to a lesser extent than CB2 receptors) and coupled through $G_{1/o}$ proteins to various potassium and calcium channels (Howlett et al., 163).

    CB1 receptors are also located in the limbic system (Mechoulam, 2006). The limbic system is involved in processing emotion and motivation and is particularly related to survival. The limbic system regulates emotions of fear, anger, and sexual behavior. It is also involved in feelings of pleasure that are related to our survival, such as those experienced from eating and sex. Two splice variants of CB1 receptors have been identified, including $CB1_A$ and $CB1_B$.

2. CB2 receptors are distributed throughout cells of the peripheral nervous system (PNS), which consists of the nerves and ganglia found outside of the brain and spinal cord. The main function of the PNS is to connect the CNS to the limbs and organs. CB2 receptors are also found on bone marrow stem cells of the hematopoietic system. This includes red blood cells and white

blood cells, which are part of the immune system and primarily located in the spleen. Small densities of CB2 receptors have recently been found in the brain, including on microglia and astrocytes, which help protect neurons in the brain's cerebellum (Pacher, Batkai, and Kunos, 410–5). The CB2 receptor can mediate the regulation of cytokine release from immune cells in a manner that helps reduce inflammation and pain.

While the above receptors are specific for cannabinoids, other endocannabinoid system receptors like TRPV1 and PPAR interact with other compounds and cannabinoids alike to regulate a variety of sensations including pain.

Ligands

Compounds that react with specific receptors are called ligands. For example, the cannabinoid ligand THC is an exogenous ligand for the CB1 and CB2 cannabinoid receptors. Endocannabinoid ligands are synthesized on demand rather than stored. Even when cannabinoid receptors are blocked by antagonists, phytocannabinoids, synthetic cannabinoids, and endocannabinoids are still able to act as ligands and induce certain physiological effects.

Gastrointestinal Function

CB1 and CB2 receptors are also expressed on neurons of the enteric nervous system, including cells of the ileum and colon. Here they modulate synaptic and junctional transmission in the gastrointestinal tract under physiological and pathological conditions. CB1 neurons were the first components of the ECS found in the gastrointestinal tract. They are expressed on cholinergic neurons, which are the excitatory motor neurons. In recent years, CB2 receptors were found on neurons of the enteric nervous system and on immune cells of the gastric mucosa. The major endocannabinoids, anandamide and 2-AG, have also been located in the gastrointestinal tract. Researchers are uncertain of the role of the ECS in gastrointestinal health, although evidence suggests that it contributes to gut motility and plays a role in preventing both irritable bowel syndrome (Sharkey) and inflammatory bowel disease (Nagarkatti et al., 1337–8).

Endocannabinoids may also play a role in regulating liver cirrhosis by acting as mediators of vascular and cardiac functions. Cannabis abuse can cause liver fibrosis in patients with chronic hepatitis C, whereas endocannabinoids can trigger blood vessel relaxation (Nagarkatti et al., 1338–9). The role of the endocannabinoids in liver disease is currently being investigated.

Cannabinoid Receptors and Brain Function

Cannabinoid receptors, particularly CB1, are most dense in the brain's basal ganglia, hippocampus, amygdala, cerebral cortex, and cerebellum and are rare in the lower brain-stem areas controlling heart and lung functions. CB1 receptors are especially abundant in an area of the brain associated with movement and postural control, pain and sensory perception, memory, cognition, emotion, and autonomic and endocrine functions. In the hypothalamus, CB1 receptors regulate appetite.

CB1 receptors are also expressed in cells that regulate energy metabolism, including fat cells (adipocytes), liver cells (hepatocytes), and musculoskeletal tissues (McPartland et al., 2014). In addition, researchers have discovered novel cannabinoid receptors (non–CB1 or CB2) that are expressed in the CNS and in endothelial cells, which are tissue cells that compose the lining of blood vessels (Pertwee et al., 600–1).

Because cannabinoid receptors primarily exist in the basal ganglia, researchers have focused on the role of cannabinoids in neurodegenerative disorders affecting this area of the brain, including Parkinson's disease and Huntington's disease. Mechanisms by which THC and CBD exert benefits include the antioxidant and anti-inflammatory effects of these cannabinoids. In addition, activation of CB2 receptors leads to a slower progression of neurodegeneration in both of these disorders. The net result of this activation is an inhibition of the toxicity of microglial cells for neurons and a reduced production of proinflammatory cytokines by the immune system cells within the brain.

NEUROPROTECTION

Besides their increased amounts in certain medical conditions, CB2 receptors have been detected in the healthy brain, mainly in glial cells, and to a lesser extent in neurons. This accounts for the neuroprotective effects of cannabinoids. It has also been noted that in brain injuries or damage, CB2 receptors dramatically increase in number (become upregulated). This is seen in many neurodegenerative disorders, including both Parkinson's disease and Huntington's disease. This increase allows both endogenous and exogenous cannabinoids to activate CB2 receptors, reducing inflammation as well as providing other physiological benefits.

Other Endocannabinoid System Benefits

Cannabinoid receptors are involved in a variety of physiological processes, including appetite, pain, mood, learning, synaptic plasticity, vision, spasticity, nausea, immune function (including a beneficial role in cancer, hypersensitivity reactions, and autoimmune diseases), seizure control, cognition, movement, and memory. The endocannabinoid system is also transiently activated under certain stressful conditions for the purpose of restoring homeostasis.

THE ENDOCANNABINOID SYSTEM IN AGING

The endocannabinoid system has been found to influence neuronal (brain cell) activity by exerting neuroprotective effects and regulating the immune system's glial cells located within the brain. Studies suggest that cannabinoids protect against age-related brain changes by their defensive efforts to foster homeostasis. Specifically, cannabinoids regulate the neurons' mitochondrial activity, reduce neuronal inflammation, provide antioxidant scavenging of free radicals, and regulate the expression of brain-derived neurotrophic factor (BDNF), which facilitates neurogenesis (creation of new brain cells). In addition, animals lacking CB1 receptors showed early onset of learning deficits associated with age-related cellular changes (Bilei-Gorzo, 3330–3332).

Cannabinoid Receptor Signaling

Cannabinoid receptors couple primarily to the $G_{i/o}$ subtypes of G protein. Once cannabinoid receptors are activated, many complex intracellular signal transduction pathways become activated. Initially, researchers thought that cannabinoid receptors mainly functioned to inhibit the

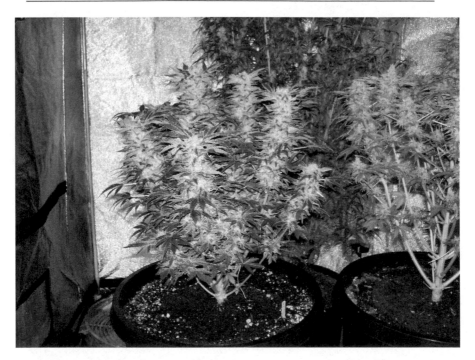

Medical cannabis growth, controlled environment (courtesy Doug Flomer).

enzyme adenylate cyclase (working through the G_i subtype), thereby inhibiting the production of the second messenger molecule cyclic AMP (cAMP). It is now known that cannabinoids can follow various signaling pathways with different end results. For example, the G_o subtype activates ion channels, and cannabinoids likely interact with other subtypes as well. Receptor density in the brain has no effect on signal coupling efficiency.

Evidence supports the important role of cannabinoid signaling in the modulation of immune function and inflammation. Cannabinoid receptors are present on immune cells. Infectious microbial antigens or other stimuli that induce immune activation modulate receptor expression. Stimulation of immune cells by bacterial toxins such as lipopolysaccharide increases the cellular levels of endocannabinoids and their degrading enzymes. Immune system modulation has been found to have both receptor-dependent and independent mechanisms (Pacher, Batkai, and Kunos, 393–4).

Intracellular signaling systems in which receptor signals converge have been found to undergo characteristic changes during aging in both neurons and glial cells. In particular, both calcium signaling and cAMP response element-binding protein (CREB) signaling, which is involved in memory formation, are diminished with age. Based on the biological effects of cannabinoids, researchers suggest that in elderly individuals, cannabinoid receptor ligands may protect against age-related cognitive deficits (Bikei-Gorzo, 3333–4). Ligands can be directly administered in the form of plant phytocannabinoids like THC, or endogenous cannabinoids can be indirectly increased by inhibiting their transporters or metabolizing enzymes. The role of the endocannabinoid receptor system in signaling is suspected of offering benefits in seizure disorders. See Chapter Six for an explanation of this process.

THC and the Endocannabinoid System

THC is the only cannabinoid found in the cannabis plant to have strong psychoactive properties, although a few others like CBN have very mild psychotropic effects. THC and most of the synthetic cannabinoids have similar affinities for both CB1 and CB2 receptors. CB1 receptor activation is responsible for psychoactive effects (which may be reduced with CBD), pain reduction, appetite increase, immune system modulation, neuroprotection, and other beneficial effects.

Ajulemic Acid and the Endocannabinoid System

Ajulemic acid is a THC metabolite that has potent anti-inflammatory and analgesic properties. Ajulemic acid is reported to bind with great affinity to both CB1 and CB2 receptors. Through this mechanism, the compound greatly reduces neuropathic pain. Given its limited brain penetration compared to other cannabinoids, it has no psychoactive effects and thus a favorable therapeutic profile (Pacher, Batkai, and Kunos, 395–398).

THC and CBD in Autoimmunity

Cannabinoids have long been known to reduce inflammation and associated pain. In one study, researchers discovered that both THC and

CBD markedly reduce the Th17 phenotype of T-lymphocyte cells. The Th17 phenotype increases in inflammatory autoimmune pathologies such as multiple sclerosis and Crohn's disease. THC and CBD were also found to dose-dependently suppress the production of the proinflammatory cytokines interleukin–6 and interleukin–10 and increase production of the anti-inflammatory cytokine interleukin–10 (Kozela et al., 1256–8).

CBD and the Endocannabinoid System

Unlike THC, CBD does not bind significantly to any of the known cannabinoid receptors (Mechoulam and Hanuš, 35–6). Instead, it interacts indirectly with the endocannabinoid system and with other receptors to produce therapeutic effects. CBD exerts its physiological effects through the following functions:

1. CBD indirectly stimulates endogenous cannabinoid signaling by suppressing the enzyme FAAH, which breaks down the endogenous cannabinoid anandamide. This, in turn, inhibits anandamide uptake, increasing anandamide levels, particularly in the hippocampus, which makes CBD particularly beneficial in neurodegenerative disorders and in reducing anxiety. Increased levels of anandamide ultimately result in greater CB_1 receptor activation (Campos et al., "The anxiolytic effect," 1407–9).

2. CBD binds with and activates other G protein-coupled receptors, including:
   a. TRPV1 (Vanilloid) receptor, which is known to mediate pain perception, inflammation, and body temperature (Lee, "How CBD Works"). CBD is a TRPV1 agonist.
   b. A2A (Adenosine) receptor, which is involved in cardiovascular function, regulating the heart's oxygen consumption and coronary blood flow. The adenosine receptor is also involved with alertness on waking and in reducing inflammation. In the brain, adenosine receptors down-regulate the release of other neurotransmitters, such as dopamine and glutamine (Lee, "How CBD Works"; Lee, *The Cannabis Health Revolution*).
   c. 5-HT1A (Serotonin) receptor, conferring antidepressant effects. The serotonin receptor is also involved in anxiety,

addiction, appetite, sleep, pain perception, and nausea and vomiting. 5-HT1A is a member of the family of 5-HT receptors, which are activated by the neurotransmitter serotonin. 5-HT receptors are found in both the CNS and PNS and trigger various intracellular chemical messages that can produce either excitatory or inhibitory responses, depending on the message's chemical content. CBD triggers a response that inhibits 5-HT1A signaling, whereas hallucinogenic drugs such as LSD produce an excitatory response (Lee, "How CBD Works"; Lee and Sexton).

3. CBD is an antagonist to the GPR55 receptor. This is another G protein-coupled receptor, dubbed an "orphan receptor" because scientists are unsure of its receptor family. Some researchers suspect it may be a third cannabinoid receptor. GPR55 receptors are primarily found in the brain's cerebellum and are involved in modulating blood pressure and bone density. When stimulated, this receptor promotes cancer cell activation and is expressed in various types of cancer. By blocking GPR55 signaling, CBD might act to decrease both bone reabsorption and cancer proliferation. (Lee, "How CBD Works"; Lee, *Smoke*, 346).

   Some synthetic stereoisomers of CBD have been found to bind potently to both CB_1 and CB_2 receptors. However, these compounds display only peripheral and not centrally mediated cannabinoid-like activity. This suggests they may act as antagonists rather than agonists at central but not peripheral CB_1 receptors.

4. CBD inhibits the reuptake and hydrolysis of the endocannabinoid anandamide and exhibits neuroprotective antioxidant activity. CBD and CB_1 receptor antagonists such as SR141716 can also reverse many of the biochemical, physiological, and behavioral effects of CB_1 receptor agonists. For this reason, it's been proposed that CB_1 receptor antagonists and CBD have antipsychotic properties (Roser, Vollenweider, and Kawohl, 208–10).

CBD and Cancer

Overall, cannabinoids are thought to cause antitumor effects by several different mechanisms. These include induction of cell death, inhibition of cell growth, and inhibition of tumor angiogenesis (blood vessel production). Cannabinoids also inhibit the local invasion and systemic metastasis of cancer cells. While this topic is discussed in greater detail in Chapter Seven, CBD's interaction with various receptors, such as inhibition of GPR55, are thought to be responsible for its specific anti-cancer effects. CBD is also able to modulate gene expression, which contributes to its medicinal effects.

Sean McAllister and his team at the Pacific Medical Group in San Francisco have shown that CBD used in conjunction with THC inhibits expression of the Id-1 gene. Inhibition of this gene has been shown to reduce aggressive, hormone-independent breast cancer cell proliferation, invasion, and metastasis. McAllister and his colleagues suggest that CBD's down-regulation of the Id-1 gene and corresponding inhibition of human breast cancer proliferation and invasiveness provides a potential mechanism for reducing metastasis (McCallister et al., 2921–3). The role of endocannabinoids as a potential endogenous tumor growth inhibitor has been suggested in a major research study where it was observed that levels of both anandamide and 2-AG were higher in precancerous colon polyps than in fully developed colon cancer. Selective targeting of CB2 receptors resulted in reduced tumor growth via changes in apoptosis, which refers to the natural programmed cell death of cells (Nagarkatti et al., 10).

Valerie Corral, the executive director and co-founder of the Wo/Men's Alliance for Medical Marijuana, reports having a client base of 600–650 patients, mostly cancer patients. Corral reports seeing most cases of cancer remission using cannabis strains with high THC, low CBD (typically strains with four to six times as much THC as CBD); high–CBD, low–THC strains; and raw cannabis extractions or the juice of whole raw plants, which provide CBDA and THCA. In cases of treatment success, she reports tumor shrinkage after three to seven months of treatment (Lee and Corral).

Clinical Endocannabinoid Deficiency (CECD)

Many conditions are attributed to deficiencies of neurotransmitters, which interfere with signaling mechanisms. For instance, Parkinson's disease is associated with deficiencies of dopamine. With the discovery of the endocannabinoid system, researchers hypothesized that because the

ECS has a greater density of receptors than other bodily systems, deficiencies in it could readily lead to disease states.

In reviewing pertinent studies testing this hypothesis, Ethan Russo proposes that a clinical acquired or congenital endocannabinoid deficiency may help to explain the ambiguous diagnostic finding in certain disorders, especially those characterized by hyper-acute sensations of pain. His proposal provides a basis for the treatment of these conditions with cannabinoid medications (Russo, "Clinical Endocannabinoid," 193–8). Later studies indicate that deficiencies in one or more components of the ECS have been observed in fibromyalgia, psychological disorders, migraine, irritable bowel syndrome, chronic motion sickness, uncompensated anorexia, uncompensated schizophrenia, and other conditions (McPartland et al., 1–10).

The influences of the ECS on the production and release of serotonin, for instance, can be used to explain the role of cannabinoids in migraine relief. Migraines are highly associated with disruptions in serotonin pathways, which can be corrected with cannabinoids. CBD, in particular, also works by reducing inflammation.

Correcting chronic endocannabinoid deficiencies may be accomplished via three different molecular mechanisms: augmenting endocannabinoid ligand biosynthesis; decreasing endocannabinoid ligand degradation; and augmenting or decreasing cannabinoid receptor density or function (McPartland et al., 1–10).

Protecting and Restoring the Endocannabinoid System

Researchers have conducted animal studies to help understand the effects of environmental agents on the ECS. Overall, they have discovered that pharmaceutical and complementary/alternative medical interventions such as massage and manipulation, acupuncture, dietary supplements, herbal medicine, acetaminophen, non-steroidal anti-inflammatory drugs, opioids, glucocorticoids, antidepressants, antipsychotics, anxiolytics, anticonvulsants, diet, weight control, and psychoactive substances such as alcohol, tobacco, coffee, and cannabis can be used to upregulate the ECS (McPartland et al., 9–15).

One example of the ways medications can help restore ECS function involves the use of acetaminophen in rats. Acetaminophen blocks the enzymes that break down anandamide, causing increased levels of this endocannabinoid. Preclinical studies also show that acetaminophen enhances the activity of both endocannabinoids and synthetic cannabinoids in rodents. These effects may be species-specific, as the results are not seen in humans.

The effects of acute drug administration are often different from those induced by chronic drug administration. For example, in rodents, acute administration of glucocorticoid steroids enhances the activity of endocannabinoids, whereas chronic exposure downregulates the ECS (McPartland et al., 5–6). Alcohol is very similar in that chronic exposure can cause damage to the ECS and other bodily systems.

Summary

The body's endocannabinoid system includes cannabinoid (CB1 and CB2) receptors; endogenous (produced within the body) cannabinoids; and enzymes. This system allows both endogenous and exogenous cannabinoids to communicate with cells throughout the body. Through this signaling, cannabinoids are able to evoke a wide range of physiological effects, including restoring homeostasis (a stable internal environment supporting general health), correcting immune system and nervous system imbalances, and fighting infections. Simply stated, the ECS regulates homeostasis and gives us the ability to eat, sleep, relax, forget, and protect.

Synthetic cannabinoids and plant extracts containing THC react with cannabinoid receptors in the same ways that our natural endocannabinoids do to cause specific effects such as stress reduction. CBD, however, interacts indirectly with the endocannabinoid receptor system. For example, by inhibiting enzymes that break down the endogenous chemical anandamide, CBD is able to increase levels of anandamide.

FOUR

Medical Marijuana

Cannabis has been used as an effective medical therapy for more than 5,000 years. In the 1930s, marijuana was a widely used drug used to treat rheumatic and migraine pain, spasms, menstrual ailments, and other conditions. With the introduction of synthetic fibers such as nylon in the 1940s, politicians deliberately lied about the abuse potential of cannabis in a misguided effort to ban the hemp plant. While this hindered research into the medical properties of the plant's individual components, in 1970 researchers at the University of California, Los Angeles, along with Robert Randall and other glaucoma patients, spearheaded the effort to resurrect cannabis as a legitimate medical therapy. This chapter describes the history and current status of medical marijuana.

Ancient Origins

There is general agreement that cannabis first emerged in Central Asia. According to the Shen Nung Pen Ts'ao Ching, the oldest known medical text, dating back to 2737 BC China, cannabis is included among drugs of the "first class," a class headed by ginseng (Earleywine, 9; Clarke and Merlin, 242–243). Drugs in this class were considered non-poisonous. Uses for cannabis in the Ts'ao Ching include menstrual fatigue, rheumatism, malaria, beri-beri, constipation, spasticity, and absentmindedness (Clarke and Merlin, 242). A warning in this ancient text cautioned that overindulgence in hemp seeds could cause one to see demons, although if taken over a long time, they could enable one to communicate with spirits (Clarke and Merlin, 242). For these reasons, in ancient times cannabis also found its place in spiritual and religious ceremonies.

54

During the second century, several new medical uses for cannabis emerged in China. Attributed to the famous Chinese surgeon Hua Tuo, who lived from 110–207, oil made from cannabis resin came into use as a surgical anesthetic, a remedy for wasting, injuries, infection, and rheumatism (Clarke and Merlin, 243). Traditional Chinese medicine (TCM) practitioners continue to use hemp seed for digestive problems and as a nutrient-rich food, as the seeds contain high levels of easily digestible protein and essential fatty acids. Hemp seeds are also used in modern TCM clinical practices for treating uterine prolapse, hastening birth, promoting lactation, and facilitating urination and defecation.

The Worldwide Spread of Cannabis

From Central Asia, hemp spread to India and from there to Egypt and Africa. The medical textbook *Athara Veda*, which dates back 3,000 years, refers to cannabis as a treatment for anxiety. Later reports mention its use as a treatment for biliary fever, congestion, digestive disturbances, depression, insomnia, muscle spasms, earaches, hair loss, poor appetites, and nervous ailments (Clarke and Merlin, 245; Earleywine, 9–13).

EUROPE

Although the medical uses of cannabis had been reported for centuries in Asia and Africa, the Roman Catholic Church opposed the plant for many years. Consequently, many years passed before the medical applications of cannabis could be fully explored in Europe. The only legal medical cures approved by the Roman Catholic Church Fathers for the people in Western Europe included wearing a bird mask for plague, setting fractured bones, cleaning burns, bleeding pints and quarts of blood, praying to specific saints, and alcohol (Herer, 191).

By the first century, the Greek physician Dioscorides had created the first known drawing of the cannabis plant and described its medical effectiveness in the *Materia Medica*, which was published in AD 65. He described its usefulness in inducing menstrual flow, relieving earaches, and alleviating muscular ailments (Clarke and Merlin, 248). A few years later, Pliny the Elder described the medical uses of cannabis, including relief from joint pain, gout, burns, and earaches, in his *Historia Nautralis*. Although evidence suggests that cannabis may have entered the British

Isles earlier, cannabis is generally thought to have first appeared in Britain during Roman times (Clarke and Merlin, 249).

By 1500, European medical publications describing the use of cannabis were on the rise. In 1532, the French physician Francois Rabelais published his famous book *Gargantua and Pantagruel*, in which he claimed that cannabis eased the pain of both gout and burns. Other European publications went on to describe cannabis as an effective treatment for mood disorders, infection, and wasting (Earleywine, 13). Thus, in 1533, while English farmers were mandated by King Henry VIII to grow hemp for its fibrous content (Lee, *Smoke*, 16), researchers began increasing their efforts to unearth the true medicinal promise of the cannabis plant.

By the early 19th century, the importance of the British hemp crop had declined due to importation of hemp from Russia and the Baltic Region. While hemp fiber was still important for ship ropes and sails, the ability to import it lessened the strain on English farmers. The search for cannabis's medical applications, however, continued to grow in Great Britain.

William O'Shaughnessy

The Irish physician William O'Shaugnessy is largely credited with the increased interest in medical cannabis in England and the Americas. In 1833, he worked for the British East India Company and the Medical College of Calcutta, where cannabis had long been instituted as a medical therapy. O'Shaugnessy investigated the medical uses of cannabis in a number of specific conditions in both animals and humans, confirming the plant's safety. In 1842, he published his medical findings in an article in the journal *Transactions of the Medical and Physical Society of Bombay*. His findings included the effective use of cannabis in relieving symptoms of conditions like rheumatism, spasticity, epilepsy, tetanus, poor appetite, mood disturbances, and nausea (Abel, 168–9).

When O'Shaugnessy returned to England in 1842, he brought with him a package of potent cannabis charas, which he gave to the pharmacist Peter Squire to make into a suitable product for medical usage. This preparation was called Squire's Extract, and it soon became the most reliable source of medical cannabis in England (Abel, 169). Queen Victoria is known to have used cannabis prescribed by the prominent physician J.R. Reynolds for the treatment of menstrual cramps (Abel, 169; Earleywine, 14). In 1845, the French psychiatrist J.J. Moreau de Tours reported on the successful use of cannabis for depression (Mikuriya). A comprehensive description of cannabis spread throughout the world, and its many contributions to medicine can be found in Clarke and Merlin's 2013 textbook, *Cannabis Evolution and Ethnobotany.*

Marijuana in Early America

In 1611, Sir Thomas Dale informed the colonists that the king expected them to grow hemp. The colonists were indifferent and soon discovered that growing tobacco was more profitable. To address this non-compliance, in 1619 the Virginia Company directed every colonist in Jamestown to set one hundred hemp plants. This provision also allotted one hundred pounds to hire skilled hemp dressers from Sweden and Poland at ten pounds, ten shillings per man if they immigrated to the new colony (Abel, 77). In 1639, every household in Salem, Massachusetts, was ordered to plant hemp seed.

In 1682, to encourage hemp production, Virginia allowed hemp to be used as legal tender. Similar laws were passed in Maryland and Pennsylvania. For more than 200 years, U.S. taxes could be paid with hemp (Kuipers, 171). Even with increased hemp production, there was a great demand by Yankee merchants needing hemp for clothing and rope. Consequently, very little hemp made its way to England.

MEDICAL MARIJUANA IN EARLY AMERICA

After O'Shaugnessy's report, physicians in both England and North America began prescribing cannabis tonics and extracts for a variety of medical conditions. In 1854, cannabis was listed in the United States Dispensatory with warnings that large doses could be dangerous and that cannabis was a powerful "narcotic" (Grinspoon and Bakalar, 4). Commercial preparations at this time were available in drugstores. During the Centennial Exposition of 1876 in Philadelphia, some pharmacists carried ten or more pounds of hashish (Grinspoon and Bakalar, 4).

THE 1860 OHIO STATE
MEDICAL COMMITTEE REPORT

Cannabis was the main topic of the 5th Annual Ohio State Medical Committee meeting. After acknowledging William O'Shaughnessy for enlightening others about the medical benefits of *Cannabis indica* (Indian hemp), R.R. McKeens, MD, described early reports of the plant's therapeutic properties plucked from the medical literature, such as the analgesic use of cannabis before amputations in prisoners on the Barbary Coast. McKeens and other members of the Ohio State Medical Committee as well as a number of international physicians and researchers then reported their personal experiences prescribing cannabis to patients.

Committee members agreed that the effects of cannabis varied depending on the plant source, Indian hemp being superior. At this time, the U.S. Pharmacopeia recognized only an alcoholic extract of *C. indica* (Extract of Hemp or *Extractum Cannabis*). The Tincture of Hemp could be made by dissolving six drachms of the extract in a pint of officinal alcohol, with the dose of 40 drops equivalent to one grain of extract (McKeens, 122–3). The alcohol extract was considered similar but preferable to the widely used hashish, which was reportedly obtained by boiling the leaves and flowers of the plant with butter.

CASE HISTORIES

McKeens reported that he used the tincture, or pills of the extract, rolled in a powder of hemp for adults with tetanus and the tincture dissolved in Syrup Rhei or Syrup Aurantii for affected children. He described the recovery of 9 out of 14 patients with tetanus using this remedy. Professor Miller of Edinburgh reported that he found cannabis an effective anodyne and hypnotic in tetanus but explained that its virtues consist of its control over inordinate muscular spasm.

Duncan, MD, of the Royal Infirmary in Edinburgh reported using cannabis as a calmative and hypnotic with no "evil" results. Mr. Donovan reported on the beneficial use of hemp, particularly in neuralgia, in his own case and that of other patients. Christison, MD, reported using hemp in many instances and observed that it produced sleep and had a powerful effect on uterine contractions. Simpson, MD, found it similar to ergot of rye in arresting uterine hemorrhage. Gregor, MD, gave hemp in sixteen cases of labor, in seven of which it succeeded well. West, MD, reported on its value in controlling neuralgic pain and recommended its use, combined with camphor, for dysmenorrhea and in flexions of the uterus. He also found it effective for controlling hemorrhages and deemed it superior to ergot of rye. J.P. Willis, MD, of Royalston agreed on its effectiveness in neuralgic dysmenorrhea, menorrhagia, tedious labor, and hemorrhage. Cannabis was further stated to reduce puerperal convulsions as well as successfully treat cases of chorea, delirium tremens, shaking palsy, whooping-cough, other spasmodic coughs, and lung diseases.

E. Dresbach, MD, of Tiffin, Ohio, received one of the first copies of O'Shaughnessy's report and was one of the first practitioners in Ohio to use cannabis on his patients. In 1856, he published an article in the *Western Lancet* expressing his confidence in its efficacy in general nervous disorders. C.E. Buckinham, MD, reported on the plant's effectiveness in acute rheumatism, initially using 20 drops of the tincture three times daily, then following the recommendation of John C. Dalton, MD, who recommended increasing the dose up to 100 drops three times daily. Other conditions effectively treated by *Cannabis indica* reported by speakers included: stomach afflictions, spasmodic asthma, placenta praevia, gonorrhea, nervous rheumatism, bronchitis, inflammatory and neuralgic pain, anorexia, laryngitis, epilepsy, hysteria, generalized spasms, and mania. In writing his report, McKeens mentioned that since the conference, he had effectively treated several patients with epilepsy using extracts of *Cannabis indica* (McKeens, 135–8).

Available Cannabis Preparations

From 1850 until 1940, extracts and tinctures of the cannabis plant were available in the United States as patent medicines, manufactured by Eli Lily, Tilden's, Smith Brothers, Squibb, and Parke-Davis for their antispasmodic, sedating, hypnotic, and analgesic effects (Earleywine, 6). Cannabis extracts were among the most widely prescribed medicines in the United States until Bayer marketed aspirin in 1899 (Kuipers, 172). The inclusion of cannabis in the U.S. Pharmacopoeia listed its use as the prime medicine for more than 100 separate illnesses (Herer, 119).

Starting in the 1860s and continuing for 40 years, the Gunjah Wallah Company made maple sugar hashish candy, which soon became one of the most popular treats in America. Sold over the counter and advertised in newspapers, it was listed in the Sears-Roebuck catalog as a delicious and fun candy (Herer, 120).

Turkish Hashish Smoking Expositions were a popular feature at World Fairs and International Expositions from the 1860s through the early 1900s. For Americans, hashish smoking became a new trend. Its effects came on faster, although the potency was only about one-third that of oral preparations. At the Philadelphia World's Fair in 1876, hashish smoking was one of the most popular events. By 1883, hashish smoking parlors were legally open in every major American city, including New York, Chicago, Boston, Philadelphia, and New Orleans. The *Police Gazette* estimated there were more than 500 hashish smoking parlors in New York City in the 1880s. In the 1920s, the NYPD reported that there were still more than 500 such parlors, far exceeding the number of "speakeasies" (Herer, 121).

By the 1890s, some of the most popular American marriage guides recommended cannabis as an aphrodisiac of extraordinary powers. There was no mention of a prohibition law against cannabis. While there was talk of an alcohol prohibition law, a number of women's temperance organizations even suggested "hasheesh" as a substitute for "demon" alcohol, which they said led to wife beating (Herer, 120). This position was reaffirmed in 2013 by Norm Stamper, former Chief of the Seattle Police Department, who wrote that "marijuana is rarely, if ever, the cause of harmfully disruptive or violent behavior" (Fox, Armentano, and Tyvert, 1).

The Hasheesh Eater

Early reports of cannabis's psychoactive effects by the authors John Greenleaf Whittier and Bayard Taylor inspired 17-year-old Fitz Hugh Ludlow to experiment with the drug, which he obtained at his favorite hangout, Anderson's Apothecary in Poughkeepsie, New York (Earleywine, 23; Lee, *Smoke*, 31). After a few low doses of hasheesh produced no effects, he took a large dose, which caused hallucinations and other adverse effects. Later settling on a moderate dose, he described the euphoria as well as laughter, dry mouth, and anxiety. Although he eventually quit using cannabis in 1857, he wrote an anonymous memoir, *Confessions of a Hasheesh Eater*, to describe his experiences and views. With perception he wrote: "Except as an antispasmodic in a very limited number of diseases, the cannabis is known and prized very little among our practitioners, and I am persuaded that its uses are far wider and more important than has yet been imagined" (Ludlow, 368). After the book's publication, Americans began to increasingly use cannabis for its psychoactive properties.

So What Happened?

In 1936, the DuPont Company got a patent for making nylon fibers from oil and needed to oust hemp fiber (Kuipers, 3). The company lobbied hard for its suppression, writing in a 1937 corporate report that ousting hemp was an important element of social reorganization (Kuipers, 4). The fall of cannabis was championed by Harry Anslinger, a former railroad inspector with no experience in pharmacology. He was appointed the first chief of the newly formed Federal Bureau of Narcotics, and his unethical political decisions almost single-handedly led to modern cannabis prohibition. Against all medical advice, the Marihuana (as it was spelled then) Tax Act was passed in 1937, and cannabis preparations were removed from the United States Pharmacopoeia in 1941. Although police began waging war against marijuana, not all law enforcement agencies were in agreement.

The LaGuardia Commission

In 1938, New York's Mayor Fiorello LaGuardia appointed a committee of scientists and physicians to study the medical, sociological, and psychological aspects of marijuana use in New York City. They began their work in 1940, and in 1944, the LaGuardia Commission released their findings in a report, The Marijuana Problem in the City of New York. This study dispelled many of the myths that had led to passage of the Marihuana Tax Act. Specifically, it found that most of the police claims that cannabis caused crime, violence, insanity, and death were completely unsubstantiated. It went on to report that the drug might have useful medical actions.

These findings were also published in the *American Journal of Psychiatry* in September 1942 by two psychiatrists who worked on the LaGuardia Committee. The psychiatrists wrote that habituation to cannabis is not as strong as habituation to alcohol or tobacco. In December 1942, an editorial in this journal mentioned the earlier publication as a careful study and described the therapeutic potential of cannabis for depression, appetite loss, and opiate addiction. Unfortunately, the journal was pressured to relax its position by the government. In January 1943, the journal's editors received and published letters from Harry Anslinger denouncing the LaGuardia report. Forced to comply after supporting cannabis therapies for 40 years, the American Medical Association established a new position, one closely allied to that of Anslinger. Behind the scenes, the federal government financed millions of dollars in government contracts to identify military uses of cannabis, such as truth serums (Grinspoon and Bakalar, 13). The government later attempted to get the reports declassified because of the medical benefits, especially anticonvulsant effects, inadvertently discovered by researchers (Lee, *Smoke*, 125).

Resurgence by the Baby Boomers

In the 1960s, large numbers of young adults, especially college students, began to use marijuana recreationally. Many students as well as their professors claimed that it calmed anxiety and enhanced creativity. They began to publish accounts of their perceived medical benefits in the form of letters to popular magazines such as *Playboy*, rather than in medical journals (Grinspoon and Bakalar, 13).

Tod Mikuriya, MD, and Medical Marijuana

Tod Mikuriya is responsible for the modern-day use of medical marijuana. He was a researcher at the National Institute of Mental Health with

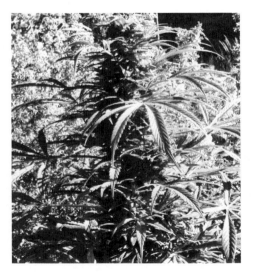

a strong interest in the medicinal potential of cannabis. In 1970, Mikuriya published an article in *Medical Times*, describing cases in which cannabis successfully cured alcohol and opiate addiction. In 1973, he edited and published *Marijuana: Medical Papers*, an anthology, which explained the safety of the drug and its benefits in the management of pain, chronic neurologic diseases, convulsive disorders, migraine, anorexia, mental illness, and infections.

Cannabis cola (courtesy Doug Flomer).

In the late 1960s, Mikuriya resigned from the NIMH and moved to California, where he continued to work as a psychiatrist. In California, he continued his efforts to legalize marijuana and began a social movement that grew into a widespread populist protest against conventional medicine and also political authority that exceeded the powers of the Constitution. Along with Michael Aldrich and Andrew Weil, Mikuriya began Amorphia. The group funded itself by selling Acapulco Gold cigarette-rolling papers imported from Spain, which were made from hemp. Encouraged by the Shafer Report, Amorphia began taking the first steps leading toward the 1996 legalization of medical marijuana in California. A comprehensive review of Mikuriya's contributions to the legalization of medical marijuana can be found in Martin Lee's 2012 book, *Smoke Signals.*

The Question of Harm

The NIH has invested millions of research dollars funding studies in an attempt to show that cannabis is harmful. Two of the major studies have been discredited, and in several other studies, changes seen in the brains of teenagers from cannabis were later shown to be as likely to be due to socioeconomic factors. Several studies, as mentioned earlier, that set out to ascertain harm found cannabis to be safe and free of harmful side effects. In several of these studies cannabis was found not only not to cause harm but to offer therapeutic benefits. While most studies have shown that cannabinoids facilitate a Th1-to-Th2 cytokine switch that theoretically could promote autoimmune reactions, cannabinoids can also suppress allergic asthma, which is primarily triggered by Th2 cytokines (Nagarkatti et al., 10–11).

Besides the other benefits attributed to cannabidiol, this cannabinoid has been shown to be effective in protecting endothelial function and integrity in human coronary artery endothelial cells. This study described the role of CBD in reducing the harmful effects of glucose on coronary cells by inhibiting reactive oxygen species; $NF\text{-}_kB$ activation; migration of inflammation promoting monocytes; and monocyte-endothelial cell adhesion (Nagarkatti et al., 11).

Discredited Studies

Gabriel Nahas, PhD, set out to prove the harm of cannabis in the 1950s. When his research studies did not show expected effects, he falsified the data. While a researcher at Columbia University in 1972, he conducted studies showing that cannabis created chromosome damage, testosterone damage, and countless other effects that suggested a breakdown of the immune system. In 1983, under ridicule from his peers who could not confirm these results and a cutoff of NIDA funding, Nahas renounced all his studies, conclusions, and extrapolations. Although in 1976 the NIH especially forbade Nahas to be funded because of his embarrassing research, he continued to receive funding until 1983. Despite the refutation of his findings, they continued to be taught for decades, perpetuating the harmful cannabis myth (Gehringer).

In 1974, the Tulane researcher Robert Heath published a study on Rhesus monkeys showing that cannabis caused brain damage. Ronald Reagan quoted this study regularly and the Hearst Publishing Company continued to publish the results in its magazines despite criticism of the study. After many requests to review the study data by NORML and *Playboy* magazine, the data was finally released. Although Heath described the monkeys as ingesting 30 joints per day for 90 days, Heath had actually

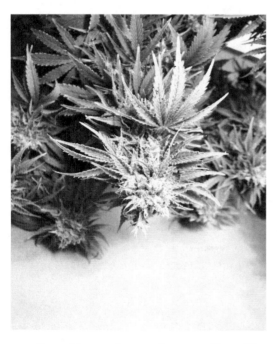

administered 63 Colombian-strength joints in five minutes through gas masks. Rather than an observation of brain cell death from regular cannabis use, the study was one of animal asphyxiation and carbon monoxide poisoning. All of the researchers who reviewed Heath's experiment agreed that the study was of no value (Murphy). Heath's study has largely been discredited by two separate controlled monkey studies conducted by William Slikker of the National Center for Toxicological Research and by Charles Rebert and Gordon Pryor of SRI International. Neither of these studies found any evidence of

Cannabis near harvest (courtesy Doug Flomer).

physical alteration in the brains exposed to a daily dose of cannabis for up to one year.

Cannabis for Treating Glaucoma

Glaucoma, a group of eye disorders characterized by raised intraocular pressure (IOP) has a hereditary component and often affects young adults. The most common form of this disorder occurs in one percent of people older than 60 and 9 percent of people older than 90 (Earleywine, 172). Approximately 300 people out of every 100,000 have glaucoma, including two million Americans, 80,000 of whom are blind (Earleywine, 173). IOP eventually damages the optic disk, which dramatically reduces vision. Glaucoma is the leading preventable cause of visual impairments and is second only to cataracts in causing blindness.

In 1970, police officers in Los Angeles noticed that suspects allegedly intoxicated by cannabis often had dilated pupils. They contacted researchers at the University of California, Los Angeles (UCLA) to see if they could correlate these findings and use pupil size as a measure of intoxication. At the time, UCLA researchers were actively studying the effects of cannabis on various biological symptoms.

Robert Hepler, MD, of the Jules Stein Eye Institute at UCLA, was asked to conduct the pupillary dilation studies. Hepler tested clients participating in the UCLA marijuana project and soon found that the police officers were incorrect. In fact, the drug caused pupillary constriction rather than dilation. Pupillary constriction occurs after the administration of several different drugs that lower IOP, including drugs used to treat glaucoma. Hepler began routinely measuring the IOP of study participants and found that cannabis induced a rapid, significant decline in IOP.

Hepler reported his findings in a 1971 letter to the *Journal of the American Medical Association* (JAMA). Over the next five years, Hepler and his assistant, Robert Petrus, continued to study IOP and found it to be reduced significantly (between 25 and 50 percent of baseline) in 80 percent of subjects using cannabis (Randall, 95). They also found that the peak effect happened 45–60 minutes after smoking and lasted three to five hours.

Robert Randall's Diagnosis and Treatment

In 1972, when 24-year old Robert Randall was diagnosed with glaucoma, the disease had already destroyed the central vision in his right eye and greatly eroded peripheral vision in his left eye. Compared to a normal IOP of less than 20, his pressure measured a dangerous 42. He was told that his vision might remain for three to five years (Randall, 96). He used the standard treatment of 0.5 percent pilocarpine and experienced blurred vision, along with a need to keep increasing the dose. In the fall of 1973, a friend provided Randall with two marijuana cigarettes.

Knowing that the appearance of tricolored haloes around a source of light occurred when his IOP rose dangerously high, he was surprised to find that 45 minutes after smoking marijuana the haloes disappeared. After experimenting and confirming his findings, he decided to purchase marijuana illegally. Later, he grew his own plants to supply his medical needs. In August 1975, he was arrested in Washington, D.C., for the crime of marijuana cultivation. Upon telling his attorney about the medical issue, Randall was told he would have to prove it.

Within weeks, Randall learned that the federal government was aware that cannabis reduced IOP. He also discovered the extensive studies of Hepler at UCLA. He visited Hepler and learned that he could expect to become blind if he remained on standard glaucoma medications. Hepler tested Randall's response to pre-rolled marijuana cigarettes provided by the National Institute on Drug Abuse (NIDA), increasing the dose until the IOP fell. Randall's physician in Washington, D.C., used Hepler's findings, which indicated a dose-related response. In addition, the Washington physician recommended that a second study be performed at Johns Hopkins University. The findings were in agreement with those of the UCLA team. The Johns Hopkins researchers also recommended against surgical intervention because of its high risk of causing blindness.

When Randall went to trial in 1976, his attorney successfully argued that his use of cannabis was a medical necessity. Following the trial, until January 1978, Randall still had to subject himself to another series of tests. He started from scratch with conventional therapies and was finally given synthetic THC pills. The pills were not as effective as whole-plant cannabis, and Randall was eventually prescribed between 8 to 10 pre-rolled NIDA cigarettes of 2 percent or greater THC content to control his IOP.

However, because Randall refused to keep his treatment a secret, in 1978 he was no longer permitted to receive cannabis even under the control of a physician. After an out-of-court settlement, Randall's access was restored and he was legally able to purchase cannabis. Randall and two other patients, Elvy Musikka and Corrine Millet, were the first three patients in the United States to gain legal, medically supervised access. By the mid–1980s, these patients were provided cannabis by the Compassionate Investigational New Drug (IND) Program. Unfortunately, because of the increased use of cannabis by patients with HIV infection, President George H.W. Bush thought the program might send the wrong message and disbanded it in 1992 (Lee, *Smoke*, 234). This action left thousands of patients in limbo and unable to legally access the medicine that worked best for them. After the program's discontinuance, the four surviving patients with legal medical access to cannabis continued to receive it from the federal government's farm in Mississippi through the National Institute on Drug Abuse (NIDA) (Grinspoon, "Cannabinopathic Medicine").

Rick Simpson

Rick Simpson is a Canadian citizen and former power engineer who pioneered the use of concentrated cannabis extracts to treat cancer. He began looking into medicinal cannabis as a treatment for his own condition of post-concussion syndrome, which stemmed from a work-related injury described in his documentary *Run from the Cure*. Just smoking cannabis did more for his condition than any of his prescribed pharmaceuticals.

Simpson's history and work is described further in Chapter Ten. He is largely responsible for the increased interest in oral ingestion of cannabis extracts to directly treat cancer, and thousands have used and improved upon his production and dosage methods to successfully combat even aggressive cancers.

California Leads the Way

In 1996, California became the first state to provide legal access to cannabis for specified signs and symptoms. Patients were required to have physician approval and to receive a license allowing them to enter medical cannabis dispensaries. In California, some people began using cannabis for children with seizure disorders. On June 4, 2011, caregivers at the Oakland dispensary of Harborside Health Center began treating Jayden David, a child with a severe form of epilepsy known as Dravet syndrome, with cannabis tincture. For the first time since Jayden was four months old, the boy went through an entire day without a seizure. "Instead of medical marijuana, this is miracle marijuana," said Jayden's father, holding up a jar full of cannabis tincture.

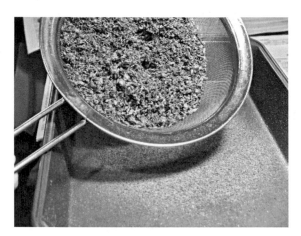

Ground cannabis (courtesy Doug Flomer).

Harborside Health Center continues to analyze and test cannabis preparations before David administers them to his son. Harborside says it helps a number of children, including Jayden, whose parents legally obtain the marijuana. His father has begun to wean him off the powerful pharmaceutical pills, which he believes have kept his son from developing properly.

Charlotte's Web

After hearing reports from California, Paige Figi, a Colorado resident, looked to cannabis as a treatment for her five-year-old daughter Charlotte. Like Jayden, she suffered from Dravet syndrome and had since she was three months old. Paige consulted two physicians who agreed to approve Charlotte's treatment as the youngest medical cannabis patient in Colorado. Paige found a Denver dispensary that had a small amount of a strain called R4, which was low in THC and high in CBD. She paid about $800 for two ounces (all the dispensary had) of bud and had a friend extract the oil. Working with her doctors, she had the oil tested and began to administer it to Charlotte. The results were stunning. After only the first dose, significant cessation of seizure activity was observed (Rabey, Steve, D8).

In need of more oil, Paige contacted the Stanley Brothers from Realm of Caring, who had developed a high–CBD oil specifically for stopping cancer metastasis. This strain, which was rechristened Charlotte's Web, has continued to keep Charlotte seizure-free. In April 2014, Paige reported that Charlotte's seizures had been reduced from 300 per week to two or three per month (Dodd, 2014). Paige and the Stanley Brothers soon embarked on a media campaign to bring awareness to the use of CBD-rich extracts in patients with seizure disorders. Many families from other states moved to Colorado to gain access to these extracts. By October 2013, 81 pediatric cannabis users were listed in Colorado, compared to four patients in 2012 (Phillips, 1).

Medical Marijuana States

As of July 31, 2014, 23 states have allowed the use of medical marijuana for their residents. In November, 2014, Washington, D.C., also legalized medical marijuana.

Individual requirements for using medical marijuana vary among the states. Each state also establishes its own rules for the growing and dispensing of cannabis products. In 2013, an estimated 19.8 million individuals in the United States age 12 or older (7.5 percent of this population) were current (past month) users of cannabis (Sacco and Finklea, 1). With the availability of medical marijuana and a general shift in public attitudes towards cannabis, more than 52 percent of surveyed adults feel that marijuana should be legalized (Sacco and Finklea, 1).

Dispensaries and Products

Individual states establish their own rules and rigorous inspection processes for dispensaries. Because cannabis is still not legal in the eyes of the federal government, harassment by federal authorities continues to be a problem, especially in California and Colorado (Grinspoon, "Cannabinopathic Medicine"). Thankfully, the latest United States spending bill, signed in December 2014, prevents the use of federal funds in the interference of state medicinal cannabis laws, effectively preventing all future DEA raids. See also Chapter Nine.

Cannabis dispensaries contain several different types of products, each of which has advantages and disadvantages. No one specific delivery method works for everyone. The type of product depends on the individual's preferences, like potency and quickness of onset, as well as his condition. Prior to the removal of cannabis in 1941, the medical literature and pharmaceutical catalogs indicated oral ingestion as the standard route (Mikuriya). While smoking is the most popular current method, vaporizers are available as a smoke-free inhalation route. Irritation from smoking can be minimized by using a water pipe, which minimizes unwanted impurities. The advantages to inhalation include: rapid onset of effects, accurate dose adjustment, fast disappearance of effects, efficient use of the drug, few metabolic effects from the stomach or liver, and difficulty in overdosing (Mikuriya).

Available products include: tinctures, extracts, oils, dried bud, edibles, topical ointments, balms, teas, and sodas. As with any drug, adverse reactions can occur, particularly when high doses are ingested. Cannabis is best used under the guidance of a qualified practitioner. As the use of cannabidiol and other cannabinoid extracts becomes more widespread, standardized doses may become more common, although the ideal cannabis doses are best determined on an individual basis (Lee and Sexton).

CBD and Acid Varieties (THCA, CBDA) in Medical Marijuana

Cannabidiol is available as a phytochemical extract of cannabis and

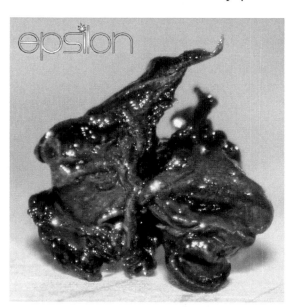

is frequently used as a form of cannabis therapy. Strains rich in THCA are also becoming increasingly popular as therapies. These products, in the form of buds, oils, edibles, inhalants, and extracts, are not found at recreational marijuana dispensaries. Hemp extracts

Isolated extract of the aromatic terpene compounds. This specimen was isolated from a hybrid cannabis strain known as GTO (courtesy Dave Mapes, Epsilon Apothecaries).

containing CBD are available online, but their source, effects, and even contamination content can vary. For optimal CBD-rich, THCA-rich, and CBDA-rich products, patients need to visit formal dispensaries. There is general agreement that CBD from *C. sativa/C. indica* hybrids works best and should be used in conjunction with THC.

Dispensaries offer a wide range of products with different CBD:THC ratios. Patients visiting medical dispensaries need to have medical marijuana cards and can apply for them with the recommendation of a doctor. Doctor's offices that prescribe medical marijuana often have the applications and other paperwork necessary to obtain a card. Today, doctors have more freedom in suggesting appropriate ratios and doses for specific conditions, but some are hesitant to go beyond only offering medical marijuana card recommendations.

Cannabis Strains with High CBD Content

Amounts of CBD, THC, and THCA can vary with growing conditions. These are representative amounts of popular strains:

1. Valentine X: a *C. sativa/C. indica* hybrid; a phenotype of ACDC with a 25:1 CBD-to-THC ratio.
2. ACDC: a 50/50 *C. sativa/C. indica* hybrid; 19 percent CBD and 0.9 percent THC. ACDC is one of the first strains used in pediatric seizure disorders. It has a fresh pine scent, and the flowers are rich in trichomes. It is especially beneficial for cancer, shrinking tumors, inflammation, pain, and associated ailments. Because it has a very low THC value, it is good for people who have issues with anxiety, nerve tremors, and paranoia. ACDC is very close to a strain called "Charlotte's Web" used for epilepsy. Its high–CBD profile also endows it with anti-psychotic properties. These formulas are ideal for people who need to work, drive, and function in the world, while providing great medicinal effects.
3. Charlotte's Web: *C. sativa*/industrial hemp hybrid; 30:1 CBD:THC ratio.
4. Cannatonic: 10.4 percent CBD and 4.2 percent THC.
5. Harlequin: C. sativa hybrid; used for pain, anti-anxiety, seizures, and inflammation; 11.6 percent CBD and 8.4 percent THC, making it more of a stimulating, energizing strain.

6. Canna Tonic (Herbal Balm): 50/50 C. sativa/C. indica hybrid with 8.1 percent CBD and 6.9 percent THC; lemony pine-scented flavor.

Summary

Cannabis has been used as a medical therapy for more than 5,000 years. Unsubstantiated reports that its use could lead to the use of harder drugs and violence, along with misguided political decisions and misunderstandings, led to its removal from the U.S. Dispensatory. In the 1970s, cannabis extracts were shown to relieve intraocular pressure in patients with glaucoma. In the following decades, the many medical uses of cannabis that were documented 5,000 years ago were further investigated and are now being confirmed in an increasing number of research studies, spurred on by a large patient movement.

In December 2014, 23 states and the District of Columbia legalized the use of medical marijuana for their residents. With an increased interest in cannabis extracts for seizure disorders and cancer, this number is expected to increase.

FIVE

Cannabis Phytochemicals and Extracts

The remarkable efficacy of cannabis stems from the hundreds of compounds present in the plant. When these chemicals work together, profound healing can occur. However, each individual constituent has its own benefits, and by producing extracts dominated by specific compounds, their therapeutic efficacy can be targeted.

While many people choose to smoke cannabis, the best way to take full advantage of cannabis compounds is through extracts. Several types of extracts with various levels of strength exist; having options allows patients to use what is best for them. It is important to take into account factors like bioavailability and peak concentrations when making these choices. The phytochemicals in cannabis and their use as extracts are explored in this chapter.

Active Phytocannabinoids and Other Chemicals

Cannabis has over 750 constituents from a wide variety of chemical classes (American Herbal Pharmacopoeia, 33). The most notable and important class is cannabinoids, a set of terpenophenolic compounds that are unique to cannabis. Over 100 cannabinoids have been identified. However, not every cannabis plant contains all these cannabinoids, and the particular cultivar directly affects the cannabinoid profile.

The two most prominent cannabinoids are delta–9-tetrahydrocannabinol (THC) and cannabidiol (CBD). Virtually all strains of cannabis have at least some amount of these compounds. Medicinal cannabis dispensaries and caregivers rely upon the ratio of THC to CBD to make recommendations to patients. The type of condition and the particular patient necessitate different cannabis formulations with higher quantities of either THC or CBD.

THE IMPORTANCE OF OTHER CANNABINOIDS

While the vast majority of scientific inquiry and public interest has been related to the two primary cannabinoids, the others are still quite important. First, they each have their own unique therapeutic benefits, which make them valuable in their own right. Perhaps more importantly, they work synergistically and mutually enhance each other's effects. A great example of synergy is how THC and CBD work together to fight glioblastoma, a rare form of brain cancer. One study found that THC and CBD, used independently, reduced viability of glioblastoma cells by 45 and 31 percent respectively (Marcu et al., 180). When administered together, viability was reduced by 98 percent, representing true synergy.

These synergistic properties extend to extracts that contain hundreds of other cannabinoids and cannabis-derived compounds. A study on prostate cancer found that a CBD "botanical drug substance" (a term synonymous with plant extract) reduced cancer cell viability substantially more than CBD alone (De Petrocellis et al., 79). Other BDS products can be designed to predominantly contain other cannabinoids like cannabichromene (CBC) and cannabigerol (CBG).

CANNABIGEROL: THE PARENT CANNABINOID

The first cannabinoid produced in the cannabis plant is cannabigerolic acid (CBGA). All cannabinoids are biosynthesized in their acidic forms until heat or time removes the attached carboxyl groups, converting the raw, acidic compounds into their neutral, decarboxylated forms. For example, in the unheated plant, THC and CBD are present as THCA and CBDA. CBGA is derived from olivetolic acid and geranyl pyrophosphate (American Herbal Pharmacopoeia, 34). Enzymes like THCA synthase and CBDA synthase convert CBGA into other cannabinoids. The particular genetics of a plant influence the relative levels of each synthetic enzyme.

As the parent cannabinoid, one would expect both CBGA and CBG to possess medical benefits. Most studies have been conducted on CBG, as the general trend of research has focused on decarboxylated cannabinoids. It cannot be assumed that properties of the acidic cannabinoids will strongly correlate with their heated counterparts, but they are all generally therapeutic in some way.

CBG has immense potential as an anti-inflammatory agent. In colitis, it directly inhibited several inflammatory markers, increased activity of the antioxidant enzyme superoxide dismutase, and reduced production of reactive oxygen species, among other effects (Borrelli et al., 1306). CBG can also inhibit COX-2, an inflammatory enzyme. Interestingly, CBGA can inhibit both COX-1 and COX-2 (Ruhaak et al., 774).

Like THC and CBD, CBG is a potent anti-cancer agent. It has been shown to inhibit numerous types of cancer, including prostate, colorectal, stomach, brain, thyroid, and leukemic cancer cells (Ligresti et al., 1375). It was a most potent against thyroid and stomach cancers, but CBD was still stronger in all categories.

CANNABICHROMENE

Cannabichromene is another undervalued cannabinoid with big potential. One of the most interesting aspects of CBC is its ability to raise the viability of neural stem progenitor cells, which supports neurogenesis (Shinjyo and Di Marzo, 432). Given this positive effect on the brain, it is no surprise that CBC also has antidepressant properties (El-Alfy et al., 434).

CBC can dose-dependently exert analgesic effects in rats by activating CB1 and TRPA1 receptors (Maione et al., 584). Since other cannabinoids reduce pain via other mechanisms, whole plant cannabis extracts seem especially suitable for alleviating pain.

Given the rising threat of antibiotic-resistant bacteria, a very relevant benefit of CBC is its ability to inhibit bacteria. The compound exhibited strong activity against gram-positive, gram-negative, and acid-fast bacteria, while also showing mild to moderate effects against various fungi (Turner and ElSohly, 283S).

Like CBG, CBC is effective against all the aforementioned types of cancer, but fell behind CBG and CBD in terms of potency.

CANNABINOL

Unlike other cannabinoids, CBN is primarily a degradation product. Over time, THC naturally converts to CBN. While producers usually aim to minimize CBN content, it still has value. First, it has potent antibacterial activity against many strains of MRSA, a range of drug-resistant bacteria (Appendino et al., 1427). THC, CBD, CBC, and CBG also have similar effectiveness against these strains. By combining the cannabinoids, powerful antibacterial results can be attained. CBN, like CBD and THC, exerts anticonvulsant effects (Karler, Cely, and Turkanis 1527).

One study using a derivative of CBN found it had potent antiemetic effects, significantly reducing nausea and vomiting in 10 of 13 cancer patients undergoing chemotherapy (Herman et al., 331).

The above study also remarked on the sedative effects of CBN, which can be adverse or beneficial depending on the situation. For insomnia, CBN seems to be a potential solution which lacks the side effects of traditional sleep aids. Many people have anecdotally reported that CBN is effective for facilitating sleep. Medicinal and recreational dispensaries alike carry extracts that are high in CBN. Unlike most non–THC cannabinoids, which are entirely non-psychoactive, CBN does possess weak psychoactive properties. This is probably due to its close relationship with THC, being a degradation product of that compound. As more applications for CBN are found, producers of medicinal cannabis products will probably look for ways to accelerate the conversion of THC to CBN.

Tetrahydrocannabivarin

Cannabinoids like THC and CBD have side-chains with five carbon atoms, called pentyl chains. All cannabinoids with this chain are derived from CBGA. However, geranyl pyrophosphate sometimes binds with divarinolic acid rather than olivetolic acid, creating cannabigerovaric acid. This acid has a side-chain with three carbon atoms, called a propyl chain. CBGV is the precursor to cannabinoids like tetrahydrocannabivarin and cannabidivarin, which have different properties than their pentyl counterparts.

Not much research has been done on THCV, but the existing research is quite promising. It shows immense potential against obesity and glucose intolerance. In experiments with mice, it reduced glucose intolerance and increased insulin sensitivity (Wargent et al.). In insulin-resistant liver cells, THCV restored insulin signaling. It is also being explored as an appetite suppressant.

THCV is an antagonist to the CB1 receptor. Therefore, it could also be used to decrease the psychoactive effects of THC or help people recover when they have accidentally ingested too much THC. Although THCV is known to be a CB1 antagonist, it likely stimulates other receptors and exerts receptor-independent effects to achieve its benefits.

CANNABIDIVARIN

Cannabidivarin does not seem to be as amazing as CBD, but its value cannot be discounted. Research indicates the main beneficial property is its anticonvulsive efficacy, which is potentially on par with CBD. CBDV was found to be significantly effective as a sole treatment against three types of seizures and worked well against a fourth type (pilocarbine-induced seizures) when combined with traditional epileptic drugs (Hill AJ et al., 1629). Unlike many such drugs, CBDV had no effect on motor function, bolstering its promise as a novel therapeutic compound.

Another study examined a CBDV-rich extract that contained some level of CBD and THC as well. In this case, pilocarbine-induced seizures, along with two other models, were reduced without conventional treatment (Hill TD et al., 679). This is another example of the superiority of whole-plant extracts containing multiple cannabinoids. THCV was also present in the extract and likely contributed to the positive effects. However, purified CBDV was of comparable efficacy to CBDV-rich extract.

CBDV and THCV were found to have therapeutic potential against nausea. Interestingly, the study was looking to see if the compounds caused nausea, as they both (especially THCV) are purported CB1 antagonists. Synthetic antagonists blocking the CB1 receptor have shown pro-nausea effects, but THCV and CBDV lacked these effects and even suppressed nausea (Rock et al., 671). THCV's appetite-suppressant effects likely derive from CB1 receptor blockade.

This is perhaps one of the greatest examples of the complexity of cannabis medicines. If cannabinoids worked through only one mechanism, then THCV and CBDV would have to cause nausea because of their antagonistic effects at the CB1 receptor. However, as the above study unexpectedly demonstrated, they do not. In general, cannabinoids exhibit bimodal effects that help restore homeostasis. The exact and numerous mechanisms by which homeostasis is achieved will take a long time to completely understand.

OTHER CANNABINOIDS

The above listed cannabinoids are by far the most prominent in the *Cannabis sativa* plant. However, there are more than 100 cannabinoids total. Many of these compounds are very similar to each other and can be grouped into categories, like cannabitriol (CBT)-type cannabinoids. Very little research is available regarding these far less popular chemicals. However, because some studies have used cannabis extracts with small quantities of many cannabinoids, it can be assumed they are exerting synergistic benefits or at least not drastically inhibiting overall effectiveness.

Many cannabinoids are metabolites, or breakdown products, of other cannabinoids. CBN is obtained by oxidation of THC and can sometimes be prevalent (American Herbal Pharmacopoeia, 36). Cannabielsoin (CBE) and cannabinodiol (CBND) are formed from oxidation or degradation of CBD. CBC turns into cannabicyclol (CBL) through natural irradiation (AHP, 36). As shown in the CBN section, these degradation products often still have remarkable medical benefits. It is important that these compounds be extensively researched along with their parent cannabinoids.

TERPENOIDS

Terpenoids are another key class of compounds in cannabis and include terpenes and modified terpenes. About 200 terpenoids have been identified in cannabis, but unlike cannabinoids, these compounds are found in virtually all plants. They are responsible for the aroma of cannabis and work synergistically with cannabinoids to facilitate healing. Although cannabinoids typically get most of the credit for the medical benefits of cannabis, terpenoids are becoming increasingly recognized for what they can do.

Terpenoids are composed of isoprene (C_5H_8) units. The terpenoid content of cannabis consists primarily of monoterpenoids and sesquiterpenoids, which share $C_{10}H_{16}$ and $C_{15}H_{24}$ template structures (American Herbal Pharmacopoeia, 37). Larger structures like di- and triterpenoids are present but in very small quantities. The potential size of terpenoids can actually get quite large as the number of isoprene units expands, but cannabis is mainly populated by the smaller compounds.

The most common monoterpenoid in cannabis is β-myrcene, which is known for its sedative and comprehensive analgesic effects. α-Pinene, another significant constituent, possesses anti-inflammatory and powerful antibiotic effects, including against MRSA (American Herbal Pharmacopoeia, 40). Limonene, commonly found in lemons, is an excellent antioxidant and has anticarcinogenic properties. Linalool is a terpene largely responsible for the therapeutic potential of lavender and is anxiolytic, analgesic, and anticonvulsant (American Herbal Pharmacopoeia, 40). It also is effective as a topical treatment for burns. Other compounds in this category include terpinolene, pulegone, and p-cymene.

While monoterpenoids typically dominate the terpenoid content of cannabis extracts, sesquiterpenoids are found in notable quantities as well. The most prevalent, and arguably most therapeutic, sesquiterpenoid is β-caryophyllene, which exhibits a number of interesting properties. It works synergistically with the chemotherapeutic agent paclitaxel, facilitating its passage into cancer cells (Legault and Pichette, 1643). It is also anti-inflammatory and anti-malarial, while exerting protective effects on stomach cells (American Herbal Pharmacopoeia, 40). Other sesquiterpenoids include α-caryophyllene, α-gauine, and elemene.

FLAVONOIDS

Flavonoids can be considered the third class of therapeutic compounds. They are less prevalent than terpenoids and cannabinoids, as only around 29 are found in cannabis. However, some have proven therapeutic effects and thus are still quite important to the overall efficacy of cannabis extracts. Like terpenoid, flavonoid is a term that encompasses multiple groups, including flavones, flavonols, and flavanones.

Unlike terpenoids, which have no unique members in cannabis, there are three cannabis-specific flavanones—Cannflavins A, B, and C. They act as anti-inflammatory agents by inhibiting cyclooxygenase enzymes and prostaglandin E2 production (American Herbal Pharmacopoeia, 40). Other flavonoids include apigenin, isovitexin, luteolin, and orientin. In general, less is known about the role of flavonoids in cannabis, but they will surely become a focal point of research eventually.

A 2014 article found that sprouting hemp seeds could induce the production of cannflavins A and B but not the traditional cannabinoids (Werz, 53). Sprouting also did not modify the favorable Omega-6 to Omega-3 essential fatty acid profile of the seeds. Therefore, hemp sprouts could be a novel anti-inflammatory hemp food product with significant potential stemming from synergy of the flavonoids with the essential fatty acids. The authors were apparently quite confident in the efficacy of this new food, suggesting that sprouts be considered for mass production and commercial development. If hemp sprouts were combined with cannabis extracts designed to be high in the most anti-inflammatory cannabinoids, then unparalleled therapeutic activity could possibly be achieved.

OTHER PLANT CONSTITUENTS

As a complex life form, *Cannabis sativa* contains far more than just the cannabinoids, terpenoids, and flavonoids. Carbohydrates, amino acids, and fatty acids, the key building blocks of life, are found in significant quantities (American Herbal Pharmacopoeia, 41). Phenols, alcohols, vitamins, alkaloids, and more are also present.

Most of these compounds have negligible or unknown therapeutic value. In cannabis extracts, many are left behind in the waste plant material. It will probably be a long time before they are properly explored, given the huge amount of work needed to understand just the cannabinoids and terpenoids.

Cannabis Extracts

Until recently, the modern medicinal cannabis movement has focused on smoking or vaporization as the chief method of ingestion. These techniques work well for symptom relief and quick onset. However, smoking is an inefficient delivery method that can irritate the lungs. It is difficult to absorb large quantities of cannabinoids through any form of inhalation. Cannabis extracts have taken prominence as the optimal way to utilize cannabis medicine, although there will always be a role for the traditional methods.

Extracts are concentrated cannabinoids, terpenoids, flavonoids, and other components of cannabis. One of the advantages extracts have over raw cannabis is an absence of chemicals with no or little therapeutic value. When a cannabis extract is produced, a large amount of plant material is left over, which is then discarded or composted. In this way, extracts are more efficient than smoking, as smaller amounts of material deliver higher quantities of the primary beneficial compounds.

TYPES OF CANNABIS EXTRACTS

To satisfy a diversity of needs, many types of cannabis extracts are available for patients. The most potent type of extract is called Full-Extract

Cannabis Oil (FECO). It has the highest concentration of cannabinoids, usually composing between 50 and 80 percent of the weight. Those looking to directly treat cancer, epilepsy, and other conditions generally need cannabis extracts with this level of potency. The color of FECO is usually black, although refinement can turn it lighter or golden. The texture is thick and viscous. It often comes in oral syringes for controlled dispensing.

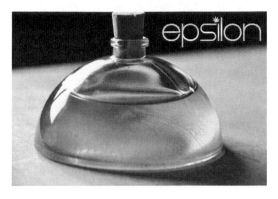

Tinctured cannabis extract made using a heat-cycling technique. This is an extract equivalent in equal therapeutic value to full spectrum cannabis oil (courtesy Dave Mapes, Epsilon Apothecaries).

Tinctures are liquid extractions made primarily with alcohol, glycerin, olive oil, or coconut oil. They are less potent than concentrated oils but can still be quite powerful depending on how diluted the products are. Drops of tincture are placed under the tongue and absorbed sublingually. These formulas usually come in small bottles with dropper caps that facilitate administration.

Cannabis can be infused into topical products like salves, balms, creams, and more. These preparations are ideal for skin conditions or localized pain. Anecdotal reports include dramatically accelerated healing and skin cancer regression from topical use. While topicals are less popular than internal methods of ingestion, they are gaining popularity as new applications are discovered.

The cannabinoid and terpenoid content of a cannabis extract depends on the strain it is derived from. Strains with high THC levels will yield extracts with even higher THC levels. Therefore, it is important to choose the correct strain with which to produce an extract. If the compounds in the strain are not well balanced or targeted, there is little hope for producing an extract that is.

How Cannabis Extracts Are Made

The concept of a cannabis extract is simple. The essential oils and constituents of cannabis are removed from the plant material and concentrated. Unnecessary fibers and biomass are left out. It is a better way to use the medicine and consistent with thousands of years of ancient herbal traditions. These traditions primarily used grain or sugar alcohols to create extracts from hundreds of medicinal herbs. In many ways, cannabis is no different.

Alcohol, which acts as the solvent, is poured over raw cannabis buds, mixed, and allowed to sit for several hours. It is then filtered and heated to evaporate the alcohol. The resulting concentrate has little to no alcohol solvent remaining and can be ingested or infused into topicals. When proper procedures and organic alcohol are used, cannabis extracts have no danger of residual solvent poisoning.

Other substances can be used as solvents besides alcohol. Vegetable oils and glycerin can be used, but they do not yield the same cannabinoid and terpenoid concentrations as alcohol. Isopropyl alcohol and petrochemicals like naphtha, butane, hexane, are effective solvents and can sometimes yield even higher concentrations than organic alcohol. However, it is difficult to completely purge these solvents from extracts, and they can pose serious threats to health. The majority of medicinal cannabis extract producers favor alcohol because of its relatively high efficiency and food-grade quality.

Another extraction technique coming into favor utilizes supercritical carbon dioxide. The supercritical state is beyond solid, liquid, or gas. Running this highly pressurized gas through cannabis has a similar effect as using a liquid solvent, but with absolutely no residue.

THC:CBD Ratios

Each cannabinoid, and particular blends of cannabinoids, is especially effective against certain conditions. For example, a high–THC formula may be best for certain types of cancers, whereas one with higher CBD would be better suited for epilepsy.

The ratio of THC to CBD is a key metric of cannabis extracts. Different conditions require different combinations of THC and CBD. While strains with very high levels of CBD and virtually no THC can be helpful for some people, a measurable amount of THC is usually needed to achieve full relief from any condition. For example, epilepsy and spasms seem to respond best to a THC:CBD ratio of 1:14 or greater ("medical marijuana"). More THC is required for cancer or pain, and 1:1 to 4:1 ratios or higher are used in these cases.

It is important to remember that everyone is different, and what works well for one person may not be effective for another. With epilepsy patients, while most are using formulas with very high CBD and very low THC, some need more THC or are even using high–THC extracts with success. Furthermore, far more research is needed to determine optimal cannabinoid ratios, so suggested ratios will likely change as knowledge develops.

THE CANNABINOID AND TERPENOID PROFILE

While the THC:CBD ratio is very important, it is only one component of the entire cannabinoid and terpenoid profile. As mentioned, the cannabis plant has hundreds of compounds. While some get left behind in the extraction process, there are still hundreds in the resulting extracts. A full-spectrum lab test will show concentrations of many compounds besides THC and CBD, such as CBC and CBG. Terpenes like myrcene and β-caryophyllene are also reported. Due to the novelty of the legal

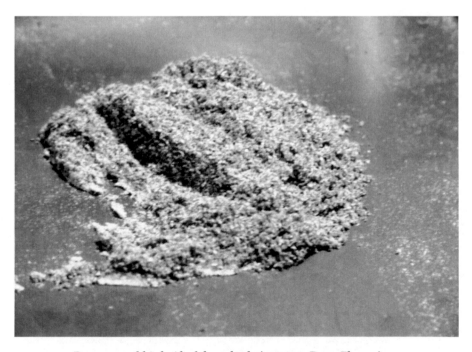

Raw, ground kief, sifted from buds (courtesy Doug Flomer).

cannabis industry, there are many compounds that laboratories do not currently test for. As cannabis medicine becomes more prominent, more labs will be willing to invest in technology to adequately measure it.

The almost endless potential mix of cannabinoids and terpenoids is what grants cannabis its true versatility. It may be found that high–CBC extracts with higher levels of linalool are best for certain types of breast cancer, or extracts with equal levels of THCV and CBDV are best for diabetes. This extensive variety is one of the underlying reasons why research is so desperately needed.

Bioavailability of Different Ingestion Methods

Depending on how cannabinoids are ingested, there are variable bioavailability rates. Bioavailability is the quantity of a drug that enters systemic circulation. Intravenous medicines have 100 percent bioavailability because they go directly into the bloodstream, but since cannabis medicines are normally absorbed through other routes, their bioavailability is lower. For example, if the bioavailability of a medicine is 10 percent, and 1000 milligrams are ingested, then the actual therapeutic quantity delivered to the bloodstream would be 100 milligrams.

Bioavailabilty within and between different methods varies substantially. THC bioavailability through smoking is between 2 and 56 percent and is greatly influenced by how the person smokes (Huestis, 1778). When orally ingested, bioavailability is between 4 and 20 percent (Huestis, 1786). This lower bioavailability results from degradation of cannabinoids in the stomach and first-pass metabolism of THC in the liver.

Methods of cannabinoid ingestion that avoid the first-pass effect have higher bioavailability rates. Suppositories are estimated to have about twice the bioavailability of oral preparations due to higher absorption and less liver metabolism (Huestis, 1793). The sublingual method, in which cannabis oil or tincture is absorbed under the tongue, avoids first-pass metabolism as well (Huestis, 1791). The cannabinoids diffuse through the mucous membrane into capillaries, where they quickly enter main circulation.

Transdermal patches are a relatively new delivery method. They attach to the skin, where they release cannabinoids directly into the bloodstream over several hours or even days. While the exact bioavailability figures have not been extensively studied, transdermal is probably more bioavailable than smoking or oral ingestion because the cannabinoids enter directly into systemic circulation (Huestis, 1794). However, because cannabinoids are hydrophobic, their diffusion across the aqueous layer of the skin is limited. This method is ideal for those wishing to sustain a steady concentration of cannabinoids. One experiment found cannabinoid concentrations were maintained for 48 hours (Huestis, 1794).

IMPROVING BIOAVAILABILITY

There are many ways to improve the bioavailability of cannabis medicines. The easiest way is to choose a consumption method that has higher bioavailability. For example, many patients and caregivers encapsulate cannabis oil in gelatin caps to facilitate ingestion. While this is a great way to avoid any taste of extract, the bioavailability suffers immensely. It is better for patients to take that same oil and let it sit under the tongue for several minutes, which will result in much higher serum cannabinoid levels.

Extracts can also be combined with other materials to increase absorption. For example, a study that combined THC with sesame oil observed bioavailability in the 10–20 percent range when ingested through gelatin capsules (Huestis, 1785). Coconut and olive oils are also patient favorites for cannabinoid delivery. Cannabinoids are fat-soluble and not water-soluble, so infusing them into fatty oils improves absorption.

Multiple administration methods can be utilized at the same time for patients wishing to maximize cannabinoid bioavailability. Vaporizing, ingesting via oral and sublingual routes, and using suppositories simultaneously can result in sustained levels of cannabinoids. This is usually unnecessary except in cases of advanced disease.

ADVANTAGES OF DIFFERENT INGESTION METHODS

Besides bioavailability, there are other preferences that influence the choice of ingestion method. For chronic pain patients, smoking or vaporizing is often preferred because of the ability to carefully titrate doses and the quick onset of effects. Patients can take one puff, see how they feel, and smoke more if needed. THC is detected in plasma immediately after the first puff, indicating rapid delivery (Huestis, 1780).

By using oral methods with cannabis extracts, higher concentrations can be achieved. Moreover, the effects of cannabinoids are extended when ingested through oral routes rather than smoking (Huestis, 1785). This is ideal for patients needing sustained relief.

As stated, some people prefer to encapsulate cannabis oil because doing so avoids the taste of raw extract. If the patient accepts the decreased bioavailability, this is fine. Using tincture sublingually is often preferred, because there is high bioavailability and tinctures generally taste better than unadulterated oil. Those wanting the highest bioavailability and serum concentrations should combine cannabis oil with coconut oil and ingest it sublingually. Although the taste can be unpleasant, the medicinal effects are worth it for many people.

Novel delivery methods like transdermal patches may revolutionize the ways in which people absorb cannabinoids. Transdermal delivery achieves many of the same goals as oral delivery, but without the taste and with even more control over dosing. Because of their novelty, transdermal patches have yet to become widely used, and more research is needed to determine their effectiveness.

Hemp Seed for Nutrition

Although they are not generally a source of cannabinoids or extracts, the seeds from cannabis cannot be discounted. Their value in supporting general health and the endocannabinoid system is incomparable. When someone is fighting a disease with cannabis medicine, it is critical for the endocannabinoid system to be healthy and functioning. Hemp seeds are a great way to ensure that the system is well fueled.

The nutritional properties of hemp seeds are excellently suited for both humans and animals. The seeds are an excellent source of essential fatty acids, protein, and fiber (Conrad, 116). The percentage composition of hemp seed of the aforementioned nutrients is, respectively, 35, 25, and 35. The remaining 5 percent is a combination of moisture and ash. Several B vitamins, Vitamin C, and minerals are also present. The protein in hemp seed is considered complete, because it contains all eight essential amino acids as well as the two semi-essential acids. Most plants do not contain complete proteins, so this is impressive. Of further benefit is that 65 percent of the protein comes in the form of edestin, which is highly digestible and stable (Conrad, 117). The other 35 percent is in the form of albumin, a different high-quality form of protein.

The essential fatty acid content is another significant benefit of hemp seed. Like the essential amino acids, these essential fatty acids must be procured from dietary sources. Hemp seed has about a 3:1 ratio of Omega-6 linoleic acid to Omega-3 linolenic acid. This ratio has been described as nutritionally optimal for long-term health (Conrad, 119). Although most people need more Omega-3 than Omega-6, it is still important to maintain balance, and having an EFA intake too high in Omega-3 can cause problems. A researcher named Udo Erasmus found that he developed thin, papery skin after using flaxseed oil for two years and that other people developed similar conditions in as little as ten months of flaxseed oil supplementation (Conrad, 119).

Two other very beneficial and rare fatty acids are found in hemp seed. Gamma-linolenic acid, sometimes referred to as "Super Omega-6," is an advanced form of linoleic acid that is more effective for lowering cholesterol than Omega-3 (Conrad, 119). Stearidonic acid, the "Super Omega-3" in hemp, is also notable for converting to the longer-chain Omega-3 fatty acid eicosapentaenoic acid (EPA) with far more efficiency than linolenic acid (Sherry). Long-chain fatty acids like EPA and docosahexaenoic acid (DHA) are what the body really needs, which is why fish oils are strongly recommended for improving Omega-3 intake.

Essential fatty acids are one of the most important components of the endocannabinoid system, so hemp seeds directly support the system that phytocannabinoids function through. The integral nature of fatty acids is demonstrated by a study that found that Omega-3 deficiency abolished endocannabinoid-mediated neuronal functions (Lafourcade, 345). If a patient is not ingesting an adequate quantity of Omega-3 fatty acids, then his health and the medicinal effectiveness of phytocannabinoids will be impaired.

The hull, or outer shell, of the hemp seed is a potent source of antioxidants. Most commercial hemp seed is sold without the shell because this makes the food far easier to consume. However, instead of wasting the hulls, antioxidants could be extracted from them. A 2012 study found that the hulls contained two compounds with high radical scavenging activity compared to extracts from flaxseed, grape seed, and soybean (Chen, 1030). It seems that virtually every part of the cannabis plant has something to offer, and full utilization of each component can impact health in a profound way.

The unique essential fatty acid profile and the high-quality, complete protein are the two standout factors of hemp seed. It is an excellent addition to any diet and may prove to be critical to fighting world hunger in the future.

Summary

Phytocannabionids are the most unique components of the cannabis plant. They are not found in any other living organism. There is significant crossover between the therapeutic benefits of different cannabinoids, but some have their own special advantages. This allows various cannabis extracts to be specially formulated for targeted purposes.

Cannabinoids work with each other and with other classes of compounds in the plant, like terpenoids and flavonoids. The best extracts maintain the integrity of all these chemicals. By choosing the right strain to concentrate into an extract, favorable cannabinoid and terpenoid profiles can be produced.

There are many ways to ingest cannabis or its extracts, and the method of intake has a strong influence on the effects and bioavailability of cannabinoids. Most patients should use methods that maximize bioavailability for efficiency and effectiveness, but there are situations where bioavailability is sacrificed for other benefits, like faster onset.

Table 5.1
Cannabinoids and Their Medical Benefits

Cannabinoid	Benefit	Synergistic Terpenoids
THC	Muscle Relaxant, Gastric Cytoprotective, Anesthetic, Antibacterial	β-myrcene, Linalool
CBD	Anti-cancer, Anti-inflammatory, Anti-convulsant, Antibacterial	Limonene, α-Pinene
CBC	Anti-fungal	Caryophyllene Oxide
CBG	Anti-anxiety, anti-hepatic carcinogenesis	β-myrcene, Linalool

Six

Medical Cannabis for Seizure Disorders

Despite having a number of side effects, drugs such as diazepam, phenobarbital, and phenytoin are the mainstay for treatment of seizure disorders by conventional neurologists. It has been known since antiquity that the cannabis plant also has anti-seizure properties. Unfortunately, over the past hundred years the federal government has suppressed medical research and use of cannabis. While cannabis was once used to treat seizures, such utility was largely forgotten until relatively recent events. This chapter describes the current medical applications for cannabidiol (CBD)-rich extracts in seizure disorders.

Marijuana Refugees and Weed

The CNN television documentary *Weed*, hosted by Sanjay Gupta, MD, sparked national interest in the healing properties of cannabis oil for intractable seizure disorders in infants and children. For many years, Dr. Gupta opposed the use of medical marijuana. He changed his mind primarily because of reports of the incredible effects cannabis extracts were having on reducing seizures that no pharmaceuticals could even marginally alleviate (Gupta). He also saw the value in CBD, a nonpsychoactive cannabinoid that had proven medical benefits substantiated by hundreds of research papers.

The *Weed* series drew attention to hundreds of "Medical Marijuana Refugees," families who uprooted and left their homes to move to Colorado, a state where medical cannabis is legal and CBD-rich oil available. These families made the move in order to provide natural plant medicine for their children. The medicine chosen was a strain of cannabis called Charlotte's Web produced by the Stanley Brothers in Colorado. The Stanley Brothers also run the Realm of Caring Foundation, which serves as a resource for families. The Charlotte's Web strain contains a high CBD-to-THC ratio, although it is far from the only such variant with this property (Young, "Marijuana Stops"). Charlotte's Web and other high–CBD oils are available in Colorado for patients who possess a state medical marijuana license. Providing cannabis oil to their child in the home state was not an option for families living out of state, as these parents would have been arrested and imprisoned for providing the life-saving medication.

STATE LOBBYING EFFORTS TO LEGALIZE MEDICINAL CANNABIS

These Medical Marijuana Refugees and their fellow activists have stormed legislatures with lobbying efforts demanding legalization of medicinal cannabis. These moms have made emotional pleas upon receptive ears. Empathizing with the stricken children and their families, legislative bodies have passed medical cannabis laws legalizing the use of cannabis oil for seizure disorders. As of June 2014, eleven states have approved "CBD-only" laws that allow for strains like Charlotte's Web, which have THC contents of 0.3 percent or less per gram, but not those with higher levels of THC (Ingold).

Charlotte's Web—Realm of Caring— Stanley Brothers

Charlotte's Web is a high–CBD, low–THC strain of cannabis. Available in Colorado, it is grown by the Stanley Brothers and provided by their Realm of Caring organization. Because of increasing demand, the Stanley Brothers are expanding production to a new facility. They also plan to reclassify their strain as industrial hemp, which would ease both growing and distribution restrictions. This is possible because the strain has less than 0.3 percent THC, which is the official legal line distinguishing hemp and cannabis (Fine). Cannabis strains available in other states with high CBD content similar to Charlotte's Web include names such as Cannatonic, ACDC, and Harlequin. For an excellent resource on the various medicinal cannabis strains, the reader is referred to the book *Cannabis Pharmacy: The Practical Guide to Medical Marijuana*, by Michael Backes.

Dr. Margaret Gedde

Dr. Margaret Gedde from Colorado Springs is a Stanford-trained medical doctor and scientist with past experience working in the pharmaceutical industry. She specializes in the medical use of cannabis with an active practice treating pediatric seizure disorders with cannabis oil. Dr. Gedde explains the utility of oil in this statement:

> In our brains and nervous systems, messages are sent through electricity from cell to cell, directing them to perform activities. With epilepsy, those signals get out of control, like an electrical storm. The research is incomplete but some studies suggest cannabinoids, when released, have a dampening effect on those signals, calming the seizures. So in kids with epilepsy, it could be that their natural cannabinoid system is insufficient [Stewart].

Dr. Gedde reviewed the medical histories of thirteen children with severe refractory epilepsy. On average, these children were treated with ten anti-epilepsy drugs without success in controlling the frequency of the seizures (Gedde). The children were then treated for at least three months with high–CBD cannabis oil for seizure control. Eleven of the thirteen children (and parents) completed interviews for the study. Four of the children had Doose syndrome, two had Dravet syndrome, two had idiopathic epilepsy, and one each had Lennox-Gastaut syndrome, metachromatic leukodystrophy, and cortical dysplasia.

Results after three months of treatment with high–CBD Charlotte's Web oil showed that all eleven children (100 percent) had reduction in motor-type seizures. Of the eleven, eight reported near 100 percent reduction, one reported 75 percent reduction, and two reported 20–45 percent reduction. Seven of eleven children achieved this reduction within the first month of treatment. At three months, five of the eleven children (50 percent) were free of seizure activity. Dr. Margaret Gedde's abstract and data were presented at the American Epilepsy Society, 67th Annual Meeting, December 6–10, 2013 (Gedde).

Stories in the News

There have been many stories related to epilepsy and cannabis in newspapers across the world. The magnitude and quantity of these anecdotal reports shows that in many cases, cannabis extracts are having truly life-saving effects for many people.

Tara O'Connell

Tara O'Connell is arguably the Australian counterpart of Charlotte Figi. Like Charlotte, Tara has Dravet syndrome. Before using cannabis extracts, she was having up to 60 seizures per day (Smethurst). Doctors said she would die within the next couple of years. She could barely walk, talk, or go to the bathroom.

As a last resort, Tara's mother began administering THCA tincture, which is the unheated form of THC. It is non-psychoactive and shares many properties with CBD, including anti-epileptic activity. Within a year, Tara's seizures stopped, she no longer needed a wheelchair, and she began improving all around. As of December 2014, she had been seizure-free for almost two years. Tara's experience inspired hundreds of other families throughout Australia, and many children are now using high–CBD cannabis extracts or THCA tinctures for epilepsy.

Cassie and Rhett's Son Cooper

The experience of a young boy named Cooper, whose last name was not given, was described in an August 3, 2014, article. The three-year-old Australian child contracted meningitis, which led to hundreds of seizures a day (Kapalos). After standard medications failed, Cooper's parents, Cassie and Rhett, turned to cannabis oil. In a short time, his seizures dropped to just two or three per day. His vision improved, along with his alertness. "Without the cannabis oil we wouldn't have our son today. We would be visiting him in a cemetery." It is not apparent what kind of cannabis oil Cooper was using, but it is likely either high–CBD or THCA in nature. As of December 2014, Cooper continued to thrive on cannabis oil, and rapid changes in Australian law should grant his family protection and better access to quality medicines.

Mia Wilkinson

A Canadian child named Mia Wilkinson was diagnosed with Ohtahara syndrome early in life. In fact, her first seizure occurred just 29 minutes after birth (Platt). The condition is usually fatal within two years. Mia experienced about 100 seizures a day. After her neurologist told Mia's parents nothing more could be done, they inquired about cannabis oil as a last resort. The neurologist agreed, given that everything else had failed and that was the only hope left. Within one day of using cannabis oil, Mia's seizures stopped and her EEG results were comparable to someone with a benign form of epilepsy. In the eight months since beginning the new therapy, her seizures dropped dramatically, with only seven occurring in that time frame.

JENNIFER COLLINS AND MADELINE LIGHTLE

A story from the *Washington Post* discussed two young patients using cannabis extracts for their epileptic conditions. Teen Jennifer Collins had been experiencing up to 300 seizures a day (Jackman). She began cannabis oil, most likely a high–CBD variety, which almost completely abolished her seizures. Jennifer said she feels a lot better, has better focus, has better memory, and does better on school tests.

Madeline Lightle, a younger patient, also experienced a dramatic reduction in seizures upon adding cannabis oil (Jackman). The oil was used as a last resort after doctors suggested removing a large part of Madeline's brain, which was considered unacceptable by the family. The cannabis medicine enabled Madeline to be weaned off all pharmaceuticals, and she experienced greater than 95 percent reduction in seizures. Her before and after EEGs testify to the profound healing Madeline is undergoing.

CYNDIMAE MEEHAN

Eleven-year-old Cyndimae Meehan, like Charlotte Figi, was diagnosed with Dravet syndrome at a young age. Unfortunately, her family lived in Connecticut, where medicinal cannabis is illegal (Leigh). The family initially got cannabis oil from a friend and began administering it to Cyndimae. She was seizure-free for three months while on the medicine. Once it ran out, the seizures returned, and Cyndimae's neurologists recommended that the family move to Maine for legal access. Upon reintroducing the cannabis oil, the child's mother, Susan, said the improvement has been phenomenal. Cyndimae has gained weight, does not need a wheelchair, and plays. The progress has been "nothing short of a miracle" (Leigh).

LYDIA SCHAEFFER'S STORY

Unfortunately, not all children are fortunate enough to gain access to life-saving cannabis extract medicine. As reported in a Milwaukee

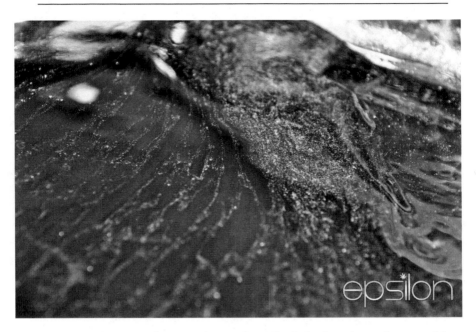

Essential oil extract of THC-rich cannabis. This hybrid strain produces a gold-speckled appearance in the yielded oil, a beautiful thing to behold (courtesy Dave Mapes, Epsilon Apothecaries).

newspaper, Sally Schaeffer fought with all her energy to legalize medical cannabis in her home state of Wisconsin for the sake of her seven-year-old daughter, Lydia Schaeffer, a victim of an intractable seizure disorder. In spite of her mother's heroic efforts to gain approval by the state legislature, it was too late (Stingl). Her daughter died in her sleep on Mother's Day 2014, before she had a chance even to try cannabis oil. This tragedy very well could have been averted had medicinal cannabis been legally available. Shouldn't every child suffering intractable seizures have the right to a therapeutic trial of cannabis medicine?

Limitations of the Patented Drug System

Perhaps the Marijuana Refugees uprooting their lives for a natural medicine is a wake-up call for all of us. Their experiences illuminate the limitations and failures of a medical system based on a pipeline of chemically altered patented drugs, foreign to nature and to the human body.

In many cases, the drugs are effective and welcome. However, in this example of intractable pediatric seizure disorders, medical cannabis oil can be dramatically more effective than conventional anti-epileptic drugs and cause fewer adverse side effects.

In medical conditions in which there is a deficiency state, replacement with the exact same molecule is the preferred treatment. This is called natural medicine. One common health issue is hormone deficiency, in which treatment with human hormones is preferable to synthetic, chemically altered hormones, since alteration of the molecular structure is known to cause cancer and heart disease. There are many more such examples in medicine where a natural substance is more effective than its synthetic counterpart.

The patent drug system has increased profits for the drug industry; however, it has corrupted the medical system, which now holds natural medicines in disdain. Since natural plant substances are not subject to the protection of patent regulation and are not profitable for the drug industry, they are the enemy of that industry. When a natural substance is found to be more effective and less costly than its patented drug counterpart, this leads to intolerable loss in sales and profit, and the drug industry must fight back against its bitter enemy, the natural medicine world.

Medicinal substances from plants and animals have served us well for thousands of years. A medical system entirely based on patented drugs is a recent aberration in the history of medicine. While there are certainly situations where single-molecule pharmaceuticals do great benefit and may even be preferred, the reliance on these medicines for treating all kinds of medical conditions is absurd. Will we see a rebirth in natural medicine and the end to this aberration in history? Perhaps medicinal cannabis is a new beginning in a shift back to nature. Let's hope so.

Paige Figi and Charlotte's Web

A remarkable development in the field of medicinal cannabis has given new credibility to its use for treating epilepsy. The neurology journal *Epilepsia* has published Charlotte Figi's successful treatment with cannabidiol in "The Case for Medical Marijuana" in May 2014 (Devinsky et al.; Cilio; Mathern et al.). The first article included testimony from Paige Figi, the mother whose administration of Charlotte's Web-derived cannabis oil stopped her daughter Charlotte's intractable seizures (Maa and Figi, 783). The child's experience was instrumental in changing Sanjay Gupta's mind about medicinal cannabis and led to her inclusion in his CNN documentary *Weed*.

Finding Help on the Internet

After exhausting all possible conventional anti-seizure medications, the Figi family discovered information about medicinal cannabis oil from a video posted on the internet. Charlotte's father, Matt Figi, discovered information about Jayden David, a pediatric Dravet patient in California. Jayden's father, Jason, had reported success with high–CBD oil for control of his epilepsy (Young, "Marijuana Stops").

Shortly thereafter, the Figi family obtained a batch of medical cannabis oil, a high–CBD strain called R4. Immediately after trying the first dose of cannabis oil, Charlotte's seizures stopped. By the time their R4 batch was running out, the Figis had met the Stanley Brothers, who provided their own high–CBD strain. After they saw how well it worked, the Stanleys quickly renamed the strain Charlotte's Web. Paige administered cannabis oil to Charlotte in controlled doses and found success in reducing the frequency of seizures from fifty per day to fewer than two to three weak seizures per month. The oil also allowed Charlotte to completely wean off conventional anti-epileptic drugs, which had proven ineffective. Early control of any seizure disorder is critical in infants, because continued seizure activity causes impaired cognitive function and at any point can lead to death.

A Facebook Group of 19 Families

A December 2013 report in *Epilepsy Behavior* described 19 families using CBD-enriched cannabis oil for treatment-resistant seizure disorders participating in a Facebook group (Porter and Jacobson, 574). Thirteen of the children had Dravet syndrome, similar to Charlotte Figi. On average, the families had found twelve different anti-epileptic drugs ineffective before resorting to medicinal cannabis. Sixteen (84 percent) of the children experienced a reduction in their seizure frequency. Two children (11 percent) had complete relief from seizures. Eight children (42 percent) enjoyed more than 80 percent reduction in seizure activity, and another six children (32 percent) noted seizure frequency was reduced by half.

Epilepsy affects approximately 50 million people worldwide, most of whom can control their conditions with conventional anti-epileptic drugs (AED). However, approximately 30 percent of these patients do not respond to traditional medications. For the 17 million refractory to drug treatment, there is an obvious need for more effective options (Zhu et al., 3).

The Endocannabinoid System of the Brain

Cannabis extracts have been used to treat epilepsy since antiquity (Kalant, 80). The utility of the cannabis plant no doubt arises from the astonishing fact that we have an entire endocannabinoid neurotransmitter system complete with receptors and endogenous cannabinoids. Phytocannabinoids like THC and CBD interact with this system to restore homeostasis. A major aspect of how the endocannabinoid system maintains homeostasis is called retrograde signaling, which is discussed further below.

RETROGRADE SIGNALING DISCOVERED

The various neurotransmitter systems in the brain use anterograde signal transmission. This means the chemical neurotransmitters travel in the same direction as the nerve impulse propagation, from pre-synapse to post-synapse. However, for the endocannabinoid system, things are just the opposite.

Dr. Nobu Kano's group at the University of Tokyo first discovered retrograde signaling in 2001 (Kano, 235; Kano et al., 309). Retrograde signaling means the neurotransmitter chemical mediators travel backwards, from post-synapse to pre-synapse, compared to the direction of nerve impulse propagation. This retrograde signaling inhibits and suppresses the release of neurotransmitters by the pre-synaptic neuron, thus inhibiting a potential seizure focus (a part of the brain where seizures begin). Given that seizures are thought to originate from overactive neurotransmitter activity, it makes perfect sense that suppressing these signals could stop seizures.

The discovery of retrograde signaling provided the impetus to investigate dysfunctional aspects of the endocannabinoid system in seizure disorders and to target this signaling as a therapeutic intervention. Since treatments related to the endocannabinoid system have shown proven efficacy, it does seem that endocannabinoid dysfunction is a major underlying cause of epilepsy.

Endocannabinoid-Related Treatments for Epilepsy

One possible treatment to enhance the endocannabinoid system would prevent degradation of anandamide by inhibiting the enzyme fatty acid amide hydrolase (FAAH). A number of studies have shown that CBD prevents degradation of anandamide by inhibiting that enzyme. Researchers have speculated that increased endocannabinoid levels may explain the clinical benefits of CBD in alleviating epilepsy, psychosis, chronic pain, and various other disorders (Leweke et al.; Bisogno et al., 845; Pertwee, "The diverse CB1 and CB2," 199).

Direct supplementation with phytocannabinoids like THC and CBD, when used in the right doses, also supports the endocannabinoid system and likely facilitates its many functions. Instead of relying solely on endocannabinoids, the system gets help from exogenous cannabinoids that make its overall job of maintaining homeostasis easier.

FUNCTIONS OF CB1 AND CB2

Phytocannabinoids from cannabis mimic our endogenous cannabinoids. They bind to and activate the endocannabinoid system in similar but not identical ways. In some circumstances, the cannabinoids may inhibit degradation of endogenous cannabinoids or even act as antagonists, blocking receptors instead of stimulating them.

For example, CBD is an antagonist of the GPR55 receptor, which is one of the ways the compound helps fight cancer. THCV is an antagonist to the CB1 receptor but, unlike other CB1 antagonists, does not cause nausea and may even reduce it (Rock et al., 671). These results demonstrate the remarkable versatility and multi-mechanism characteristics of phytocannabinoids, even when they are acting as antagonists.

ENDOCANNABINOIDS IN SEIZURE DISORDERS

In 2008, Dr. Anikó Ludányi published a study in the *Journal of Neuroscience* showing that patients suffering from temporal lobe epilepsy have a dysfunctional endocannabinoid system (Ludányi et al., 2976). Logically, it makes sense that restoring proper function to the endocannabinoid system could have therapeutic benefits. Dr. Ludányi writes:

> Endocannabinoid signaling is a key regulator of synaptic neurotransmission throughout the brain. Compelling evidence shows that its perturbation leads to development of epileptic seizures, thus indicating that endocannabinoids play an intrinsic protective role in suppressing pathologic neuronal excitability [Ludányi et al., 2976].

The doctor's study analyzed postmortem brain tissue from the hippocampus in temporal lobe epilepsy patients. Comparison was made to normal brains, which served as controls. He found that the CB1 cannabinoid receptor messenger RNA was reduced to one-third that of normal brains. In addition, there was a 60 percent reduction in the level of the enzyme responsible for the endocannabinoid 2-AG's synthesis.

Using immune-labeling techniques, Dr. Ludányi found reduced density of CB1 receptors in the epileptic focus in the dentate gyrus of the hippocampus. Electron microscopy of the dentate gyrus revealed pronounced reduction in axon terminals. Dr. Ludányi concluded:

> Downregulation of CB(1) receptors along with other components of the endocannabinoid system may facilitate increased network excitability.... These findings show that a neuroprotective machinery involving endocannabinoids is impaired in [the] epileptic human hippocampus [Ludányi et al., 2976].

The Nervous System Basics, Neurotransmitters, and the Synapse

Our nervous system consists of nerve cells, which have long slender fibers called axons. Communication of one nerve cell with another takes place at the specialized unit called the synapse, the point of contact between one axon and the next, represented by a narrow slit-like space between the two nerve units. This narrow space, known as the synaptic cleft, is where chemical neurotransmitters are released and sent across to the post-synaptic neuron, triggering a new electrical pulse in the next axon. Thus the nerve impulse propagates along its path in the brain. Through mapping of the fiber tracts in the brain, it is known that many circuitous loops exist, in which pulses feed back to their origin. Normally these returning pulses are attenuated by the dampening effect of

99

the endocannabinoid system. Should the system be defective, as shown above, these feedback signals are amplified with each turn of the circuit. Eventually a threshold is exceeded, triggering a generalized electrical discharge called a seizure. If you observe a patient having a seizure, you may notice uncontrollable rhythmic movements of the arms, legs, face, and mouth, with biting of the tongue and froth appearing at the oral cavity. A catastrophic outcome from such activity is respiratory or cardiac arrest, which can be fatal. In infants, intractable seizure activity may lead to cognitive and behavioral problems (Van Rijckevorsel, 227; Besag, 119).

NUCLEAR MELTDOWN

The events leading to a seizure may be compared to chain reaction in a nuclear reactor power plant. In the worst-case scenario, the chain reaction leads to a meltdown of the reactor core and potentially nuclear detonation. To prevent such a catastrophe, the reactor is controlled by insertion of graphite rods into the reactor core, which soak up excess neutrons and slow the reaction. This controls the reaction and prevents the reactor from overheating. These graphite rods are to the nuclear reactor as our endocannabinoid system is to our brains: a dampening mechanism for reducing excitability and inhibiting seizure activity.

Endocannabinoid System Prevents Seizure Activity

As mentioned above, the function of the endocannabinoid system in the brain is to dampen synaptic feedback loops, thus preventing seizure activity. This is achieved largely through retrograde feedback, where endocannabinoids traveling upstream from the post-synaptic neuron tell the pre-synaptic neuron to stop releasing neurotransmitters (Alger, 169; Lutz, "Physiological"; Monory et al., 455).

Studies show that endocannabinoid levels are strongly elevated after seizure activity in experimental models of induced epilepsy, indicating attempted suppression of the seizure focus. In addition, endogenous cannabinoids that bind to and activate pre-synaptic CB1 receptors, primarily 2-AG, prevent epileptic seizures in neuron cell culture and animal models. Even synthetic molecules designed to bind to the CB1 receptor will dampen seizure activity (Deshpande et al., 52; Goffin, Paesschen, and Laere, 1033; Welty, Luebke, and Gidal, 250).

Making the Case with Basic Science

In his 2013 article, Dr. Hofmann laments the insufficient number and quality of human studies to establish the case for CBD as a treatment for epilepsy (Hofmann and Frazier, 43). However, he says the basic evidence is compelling. The CB1 cannabinoid receptor is highly expressed in the central nervous system, almost exclusively at the pre-synaptic neuron. When the CB1 receptor is activated by endogenous cannabinoids, there is inhibition of synaptic transmission, typically via action on voltage-gated calcium or potassium channels. Dr. Hofmann says there is considerable basic evidence for the following:

1. The endocannabinoid system inhibits excitability of neurons in the brain.
2. The endocannabinoid system is altered by epileptic seizures.
3. Using drugs to modulate the endocannabinoid system reduces seizure activity in various animal models. Dr. Hofmann says:

The current research demonstrates obvious changes to CB1R expression in epilepsy.... Current data broadly suggest the possibility that CB1R expression tends to be up-regulated at GABAergic synapses and down-regulated at glutamatergic synapses in epilepsy ... noteworthy in that both of these changes to CB1R expression could plausibly contribute to reduced seizure threshold in epileptic tissue [Hofmann and Frazier 43].

INHIBITING OR INDUCING SEIZURE ACTIVITY

Dr. Deshpande's 2009 study of hippocampal neurons in cell culture showed anandamide and 2-AG inhibited status epilepticus in a dose-dependent manner. Conversely, treating the neurons with a CB1-blocking drug (such as AM251) potentiated the seizure activity (Deshpande et al., 52). Similar observations were made in animal models, in which treatment with CB1-blocking drugs, or genetic manipulation of the CB1 receptor, induced seizures. In severe long-standing epilepsy, the protective endocannabinoid signaling pathway is disrupted, accounting for reduced seizure threshold and increased neuronal damage.

NOISE CONTROL

In a noisy room, one can turn down the volume on a hearing aid, sparing damage to hearing. Similarly, the endocannabinoid system enables neurons to dampen and reduce the amplitude of received signals, thus providing protection from over-excitability.

ANIMAL STUDIES, DR. WALLACE

Dr. Wallace reported in the 2003 *Journal of Pharmacology* that the endogenous cannabinoid system regulates seizure frequency and duration in an animal model of temporal lobe epilepsy (Wallace et al., "The endogenous," 129). During chemically induced seizures, the amount of 2-AG increased within the hippocampus, an important brain structure linked to long-term memory formation. In addition, molecular analysis showed increased CB1 receptor protein expression in the CA regions of the epileptic hippocampus. These observations suggest that the endocannabinoid system is intimately linked to regulation of neuronal signals in the hippocampus.

Early Studies

Mechoulan and Cunha conducted early studies on epilepsy in humans in 1980 (Cunha et al., 175). The results were promising; the small number of study subjects is the primary criticism. In this study, 200–300 mg of CBD was administered daily, and seven of eight treated patients experienced significant improvements, including four who became almost seizure-free. Unfortunately, after the positive results were seen, no follow-up was conducted to see if the success could be replicated in a larger patient population.

A Search for the Active Ingredient

There are more than 100 different cannabinoids in the cannabis plant. However, the two most studied are the two most prominent compounds, THC and CBD. The latter in particular has been studied for its role in potentially combating epilepsy (Jones et al., "Cannabidiol exerts," 344).

In a 2012 study by Dr. Jones using CBD in differing animal models of drug-induced seizures, the author concluded:

> When combined with a reported absence of psychoactive effects, this evidence strongly supports CBD as a therapeutic candidate for a diverse range of human epilepsies.... CBD acts in a CB(1) receptor-independent manner, to inhibit epileptiform activity in vitro and seizure severity in vivo [Jones et al., "Cannabidiol displays," 569].

Mechanism of Action Remains Elusive

CBD is known to have a potent anticonvulsant effect in animal models and human studies. However, as of December 2014, the precise mechanism of action remains unknown. What is known is that CBD exerts its direct effects independent of the CB1 receptor. Most experts agree that CBD's effects are mediated by reduced degradation of endogenous cannabinoids, allowing for increased availability of anandamide and 2-AG at the synaptic clefts (Leweke et al.; Bisogno, 845; Pertwee, 199).

Cannabidivarin: Another Promising Cannabinoid

In 2012, Dr. Hill published a study using the cannabinoid CBDV in epilepsy with promising results. In a mouse model of chemically induced seizures, he found CBDV to be effective as an anticonvulsant over a range of different animal seizure models (Hill et al., 1629).

Receptor-Independent and Dependent Mechanisms of THC and CBD

Dr. Wallace studied the role of CB1 receptors in epilepsy, finding that "activation of the CB1 receptor has proven to dampen neurotransmission and produce an overall reduction in neuronal excitability" (Wallace et al., "Assessment," 51). He also concluded that "anticonvulsant effects of THC and the drug WIN 55 are cannabinoid CB1 receptor-mediated while the anticonvulsant activity of cannabidiol is not."

A Balance Between Inhibition and Excitation

In the brain there is a balance between inhibitory and excitatory neurotransmission. If the intensity of excitatory transmission exceeds a certain threshold, then epileptic seizures can occur. Dr. Lutz reported in 2004 that CB1 receptors expressed on excitatory (glutamatergic) neurons mediate the anticonvulsive activity of endocannabinoids (Lutz, "On-demand," 1691).

Reporting in 2008 on an electro-shock mouse model of seizures, Dr. Naderi evaluated the interactions between cannabinoid compounds and the anticonvulsant drug diazepam (Valium) (Naderi et al., 1501). He found that the effects of cannabinoids on epilepsy were dependent upon the responsiveness of gabaminergic and glutamatergic neurotransmission. The antiepileptic effects of cannabinoids were explained by inhibition of excitatory glutamate neurotransmission. Yet, Dr. Naderi found an antagonistic interaction with diazepam due to cannabinoid inhibition of the gabaginergic system.

In 2006, Dr. Pál Pacher studied the endocannabinoid system in a rat model of drug-induced epilepsy. CB1 receptor agonists were more effective as anticonvulsants than commonly used anticonvulsant drugs such as Dilantin and Phenobarbital (Pacher, Bátkai, and Kunos, 389).

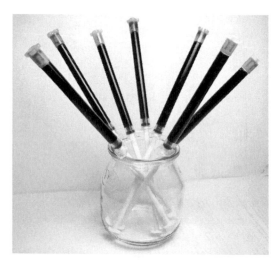

Syringes with cannabidiol oil for oral, topical or suppository use (courtesy Doug Flomer).

Summary

The endocannabinoid system has been implicated in regulating neuronal communication via post-synaptic feedback. Endocannabinoids traveling upstream attach to pre-synaptic CB1 receptors and inhibit further neurotransmission. Epileptic seizures emerge when this mechanism fails and excitatory neurotransmission becomes uncontrolled.

Phytocannabinoids like

THC and CBD have been shown to have anti-epileptic activity in cell and animal studies, although they operate through different mechanisms. The few human results that exist strongly suggest that these effects translate to people.

Although the number and quality of human clinical studies on the use of CBD and other cannabinoids in epilepsy are considered "inconclusive" by mainstream medicine, the basic science is very strong, and one may predict an important role for cannabinoid medicine as a treatment for seizure disorders.

Seven

Medical Cannabis for Cancer and Pain

In 1974, scientific evidence emerged suggesting cannabinoids could potentially treat cancer. The first study showed THC to be effective against a type of lung cancer known as Lewis lung adenocarcinoma. Since then, studies have shown THC, CBD and other cannabinoids effective as anti-cancer agents. The cannabinoids utilize existing cell machinery and pathways to cause cancer cells to undergo programmed cell death, also called apoptosis. When this body of research is examined, it becomes clear that cannabinoids are destined to play an important role in cancer treatment.

Many studies also demonstrate how cannabinoids can treat several different types of pain without the traditional side effects of opiates. Unlike cannabis for cancer, which has relatively few clinical trials, studies of cannabis to alleviate pain boasts dozens of clinical trials with positive results. Neuropathic pain and fibromyalgia respond especially well to cannabis medicine. Metastatic cancer may destroy tissues and cause severe pain which may also respond to medicinal cannabis, thus offering a more comprehensive solution. The use of cannabis extracts in cancer and pain is the focus of Chapter Seven.

What Makes a Cancer Cell? The Eight Hallmarks of Cancer

Before we discuss the anti-cancer effects of cannabis, we must first examine cancer cells and understand how they differ from normal cells. Perhaps the most seminal article summarizing the current state of our knowledge on cancer comes from Dr. Douglas Hanahan and Dr. Robert Weinberg. Their article "The Hallmarks of Cancer" was published in 2000 and revised in 2011 (Hanahan and Weinberg, 646). The original version has six hallmarks, while the revised version added two more.

NUMBER ONE:
SELF-SUFFICIENCY IN GROWTH SIGNALS

One of the primary hallmarks of cancer is that the cancerous cells can produce their own chemicals to drive tumor growth. Signaling factors such as VEGF (vascular endothelial growth factor) bind to cell membrane receptors, which then activate the MAPk/Erk signaling pathway. This pathway activates or "turns on" genetic expression for cell growth in the nuclear DNA. Normally, adult cells stop growing and spend most of their time in a quiescent phase doing their specialized jobs as "worker bees" in the hierarchy of the organism. In order to leave the dormant state and start growing and replicating, the cell requires growth factors. This growth-factor requirement is a limit that prevents normal cells from growing beyond their normal point. The mission of the cancer cell is to grow uncontrollably, but without growth factors, this is not possible. However, the cancer cell has bypassed this checkpoint by either generating its own growth factors or eliminating the need for them, usually by mutating the Ras protein into a "permanent on" signal.

NUMBER TWO:
INSENSITIVITY TO ANTIGROWTH SIGNALS

Antigrowth signaling proteins outside normal cells tell them to stop growing and replicating. Cancer cells have mutations in these cell signaling proteins that normally provide checkpoints in the cell cycle. The cells become insensitive to antigrowth signals and continue to divide. The combination of antigrowth-factor resistance and self-production of pro-growth compounds explains why cancers are so hard to eliminate.

NUMBER THREE: EVADING APOPTOSIS

Evading apoptosis, programmed cell death, is perhaps one of the most important of the hallmarks of cancer. When normal cells become damaged, they are programmed to kill themselves for the benefit of the organism. In fact, ten million of our own cells undergo apoptosis (derived from the Greek word for "falling away") every day (Elmore, 495). Cancer cells no longer concern themselves with the health of their host and prevent themselves from undergoing apoptosis.

Strictly speaking, cannabinoids do not actually "kill" anything. Rather, they serve as messengers that trigger cell-signaling pathways leading to apoptosis. This is a normal part of the cell cycle and a mechanism for destroying unwanted or damaged cells. The body even has some defense mechanisms to encourage apoptosis in cancer cells, but the failure of these mechanisms leads to cancer's uncontrolled growth. More on the critical process of apoptosis is discussed after the other hallmarks of cancer.

Number Four: Limitless Replication Potential

Normal cells have a well-defined life cycle. They start out as primitive stem cells and then differentiate into predestined specialized cell types (liver cells, muscle cells, nerve cells, light receptor cells, red blood cells, etc.). Once differentiated, these mature cells have a limited life span, replicating about 50 to 60 times. Cell replication is limited by the Hayflick Limit, a phenomenon named after Leonard Hayflick, who discovered it. During the life span of a cell, there is an accumulation of oxidative damage and loss of function. Oxidative damage to cell organelles is a normal side effect of mitochondrial energy production. Once cells become dysfunctional, internal mechanisms signal that it is time for programmed cell death. This end-of-life event for the cell is called "cell senescence."

The Cell Time Clock: The Telomere

The time clock, which controls the Hayflick Limit, is located at the ends of a chromosome and is called the telomere. Telomeres are regions of repetitive nucleotide sequences that protect chromosomes and facilitate replication. They shorten slightly every time cell division takes place. Similar to a candle burning down, telomeres eventually become too short and then signal the cell to enter senescence and ultimately programmed cell death.

For cancer cells, the Hayflick Limit does not apply, as they will replicate indefinitely. But how do cancer cells avoid this limit, given that their telomeres shorten after division? Their ability to regenerate telomeres by making an enzyme called telomerase is the answer. This allows them to escape cell senescence and the Hayflick Limit. They are now freed from control and can replicate as immortal cells indefinitely. However, the price for immortality is continuous accumulation of genetic damage, which is visible upon microscopic examination of cancer cells.

NUMBER FIVE: SUSTAINED ANGIOGENESIS

A growing mass of cancer cells has a voracious appetite for nutrition, mostly in the form of glucose. These nutrients can only be supplied by blood flow; therefore, cancers need new blood vessels to provide nourishment. Signaling molecules such as vascular endothelial growth factor (VEGF) stimulate the formation of blood vessels. In normal organisms, angiogenesis is a carefully controlled physiologic event found in wound healing, embryogenesis, ischemia, and inflammation. On the other hand, angiogenesis induced by tumors tends to be uncontrolled. This results in the well-known hypervascular "tumor blush" visible on contrast-enhanced imaging techniques like CAT or MRI scans. Tumor blush is a telltale sign of a growing malignancy.

NUMBER SIX:
TISSUE INVASION AND METASTASES

A growing lump detected somewhere in the body is bad enough. Even worse, cancer cells have the perfidious ability to spread elsewhere and grow satellite masses in distant locations. This is called metastatic disease and is usually a poor prognostic indicator. The production of proteolytic enzymes, which dissolve the extracellular matrix, called matrix metalloproteineases, allows cancer cells to become locally invasive. This frightful ability of the cancer cell to invade is a feature shared by the trophoblast cell of the placenta and is the basis for the Trophoblast Theory of Cancer, originally proposed in 1906 by the Scottish embryologist John Beard (Beard, 140). For more than 100 years, the Trophoblast Theory was largely ignored by the scientific community until recent advances in molecular biology have indeed confirmed that cancer cells share many of the molecular pathways and circuits of the trophoblast (Ferretti et al., 121).

NUMBER SEVEN:
ABNORMAL METABOLIC PATHWAYS

Abnormal metabolic pathways and the Warburg Effect were featured in the 2011 update of the Trophoblast Theory. A primary difference between healthy and cancerous cells relates to the Warburg Effect, first described in 1924 by Dr. Otto Warburg. He observed that cancer cells shift energy production from normal oxidative respiration to glycolysis, a more primitive state similar to a fermenting yeast cell, in which glucose is converted to energy with lactic acid as a byproduct (Ward and Thompson, 297).

Normal mammalian cells use oxygen to produce energy through oxidative phosphorylation, taking place in the mitochondrial electron transport chain. Normal cells revert to glycolysis as an alternate pathway under conditions of oxygen deprivation. For cancer cells, however, mitochondrial energy production is locked into the glycolysis pathway, even in the presence of plentiful oxygen.

NUMBER EIGHT: EVADING THE IMMUNE SYSTEM

Isolated cancer cells normally persist throughout the body, and it is only when their growth is uncontrolled that tumors arise. The immune system normally locates and digests cancerous cells before malignancy occurs. However, some cancers are especially good at avoiding the immune system, or the system is too damaged to contain the growth. That is why having a strong immune system is critical to both preventing and fighting cancer.

Various Roles of Apoptosis

As stated, cells are programmed to undergo apoptosis when they reach a certain level of damage or approach the Hayflick Limit. Even cells that have become cancerous have internal means of apoptosis being restored. When this regulation is impeded, cancer cell proliferation overwhelms the body and tumors form, with metastasis the inevitable final step if anti-cancer therapies are not employed.

Remember those old spy movies. Just before being sent off on a new mission, the secret agent was handed a cyanide pill to be used in the event of capture. Committing suicide was preferable to torture and disclosure of secret information to the enemy. All of our cells have this "suicide pill" ready for use when the time comes. If activated, molecular programs hardwired inside the cell trigger an irreversible cascade culminating in organized cell death. Cannabinoids like THC and CBD, as well as other exogenous and endogenous compounds, trigger cancer cells to die by suicide.

EMBRYOLOGY RELIES ON APOPTOSIS

Embryologic development relies on apoptosis to remove unwanted cells to form appendages, organs, and tissue layers. An example is removal of the tadpole tail to form a frog. The tail cells are "removed" by undergoing apoptosis. Another example is the webbing between the fingers of a human embryo. These cells are also removed by apoptosis to form well-defined fingers. In disease states, there may be disruption in the cellular machinery or signaling pathways that control apoptosis. Excessive apoptosis may cause neurodegenerative disease, and insufficient apoptosis may cause cancer (Elmore, 495).

APOPTOSIS VS. NECROSIS

Apoptosis is characterized by cell shrinkage and preservation of the cell membrane. This keeps its content contained as the cell goes through organized dissolution and digestion. Apoptosis is distinguished from necrosis, a more brutal form of cell death caused by toxic injury from chemotherapy. Necrotic cells typically show cytoplasmic swelling and rupture of the cell membrane, with release of cellular debris into the surrounding tissues, which evokes an inflammatory response. A quote from *Molecular Biology of the Cell* explains this difference:

> Cells that die as a result of acute injury typically swell and burst. They spill their contents all over their neighbors—a process called cell necrosis—causing a potentially damaging inflammatory response. By contrast, a cell that undergoes apoptosis dies neatly, without damaging its neighbors. The cell shrinks and condenses. The cytoskeleton collapses, the nuclear envelope disassembles, and the nuclear DNA breaks up into fragments. Most importantly, the cell surface is altered, displaying properties that cause the dying cell to be rapidly phagocytosed, either by a neighboring cell or by a macrophage, before any leakage of its contents occurs. This not only avoids the damaging consequences of cell necrosis but also allows the organic components of the dead cell to be recycled by the cell that ingests it [Alberts et al.].

THE ROLE OF MITOCHONDRIA IN APOPTOSIS

While there are many pathways leading to apoptotic cell death, most of them converge on the mitochondria, little oval organelles within the cell that are involved in energy production. Signaling proteins (Bax) attach to the mitochondrial membrane to induce release of cytochrome C, which binds to a protein called Apaf–1. This induces formation of the apoptosome, a seven-spoke wheel protein molecule, which activates the caspase cascade, an irreversible event leading to cell death.

The p53 Gene: "Guardian of the Genome"

Our DNA may be damaged by environmental chemicals, irradiation, or even by oxidation generated by normal cellular energy production. The p53 gene, dubbed "Guardian of the Genome," detects DNA damage in the nucleus. In the event of DNA damage, the cell cycle is arrested to initiate DNA repair. If the damage exceeds the capacity for repair, then the p53 gene triggers apoptosis via the death-signal protein Bax. A common method cancer cells use to evade apoptosis is to harbor a mutation in the p53 gene, rendering it non-functional. Roughly half of all cancers have mutations in this gene.

What Causes Cancer?

There are many potential reasons cancers arise, but the causes usually boil down to DNA damage. Carcinogenic chemicals are a key contributor to cancer, as they cause oxidative damage to nuclear and mitochondrial DNA. When the DNA repair mechanisms are overwhelmed, normal cells are transformed into cancer cells. Also, an individual's genetic background can significantly influence whether he gets cancer or not.

Mitochondria are critical to both the development and resolution of cancer. Given that they are the energy production centers of the cell and that cancer cells produce energy differently, it makes sense that mitochondria would be intimately involved. Indeed, cell mitochondria were found to be defective or even absent when cancer cells were analyzed with electron microscopy (Seyfried and Shelton, 269). The mitochondria of cancer cells are essentially reprogrammed to serve as "biosynthetic organelles" whose main job is to grow the tumor mass by consuming large amounts of glucose (Ward and Thompson, 297).

How Does Cannabis Kill Cancer Cells?

As described previously, the cancer cell is a mutated, primitive cell exhibiting eight hallmarks, one of which is the ability to evade apoptosis. If we could somehow restore and trigger the pathways for programmed cell death in cancer cells, while sparing normal cells, we would have an exceptional cancer treatment. This is the beauty of natural plant substances such as the cannabinoids THC and CBD, which instruct cancer cells but not healthy ones to undergo apoptosis.

There is an abundance of research illuminating how cannabis fights cancer. Unfortunately, the vast majority of research has been done using only cell and animal models. While preclinical evidence of this sort does not always translate to humans, cannabinoids are an exception. Several aspects of preclinical and animal research suggest that the results would translate very well to humans. Moreover, the vast amount of anecdotal evidence indicating complete remissions in cancer patients using cannabis extracts shows the need for more clinical trials. Cannabidiol has also received approval for the treatment of glioma.

Basic Science Methods

The basic science of cannabis cancer research involves studying cancer cells in culture by treating them with cannabinoids (mainly THC and CBD) and other agents. After this, the cancer cells are studied to determine the effect. A second method is the in-vivo animal study, usually done with mice injected with cancer cells (called a xenograft) and then treated with cannabis agents. The mice are observed and then sacrificed so that their organs can be studied.

Brain Cancer

It is well known that cannabinoids can cross the blood-brain barrier, as this is how psychoactive effects are conferred. Therefore, the compounds may offer especially potent treatments for a variety of brain cancers, and the research surrounding glioma in particular is especially strong.

Dr. Manuel Guzmán and the Cannabinoid Signaling Group in Madrid Spain

Dr. Manuel Guzmán has devoted his career to the anti-cancer activity of phytocannabinoids such as THC and CBD. In an editorial in 2012, Dr. Guzmán states that the anti-cancer effects of cannabinoids are due to their ability to induce apoptosis in cancer cells. In addition, Dr. Guzmán cites animal experiments showing that cannabinoids inhibit angiogenesis (new vessel growth) in cancerous tissue, block invasion of surrounding tissues, and prevent metastatic spread of cancer cells (Velasco, Sánchez, and Guzmán, 436).

Accumulation of Ceramide in Glioma Cells

Much of Dr. Guzmán's work has focused on the study of brain cancers, specifically gliomas, which arise from glial cells. Forms include glioblastoma, astrocytoma, and optic nerve glioma. These are perhaps the most devastating of all cancer types, tending to be very aggressive, with high recurrence rates after chemotherapy and radiation therapy. Prognosis for this type of cancer is unusually poor. Senator Edward "Ted" Kennedy succumbed to glioblastoma 15 months after diagnosis. Median survival for glioblastoma was extended from 12.2 months to 14.6 months after introduction of a new drug in 2005 called temozolomide.

Dr. Guzmán reports that THC and other cannabinoids induce programmed cell death in glioma cell lines grown in culture. They do this by activating CB1 or CB2 receptors, which leads to intracellular accumulation of the apoptosis-signaling molecule ceramide (Velasco, Sánchez, and Guzmán, 436). Ceramide accumulation causes structures called autophagosomes to attach to the mitochondria, which then undergo mitophagy (they "eat themselves"). Autophagosomes are unique double-membrane vesicles whose presence indicates the cells are undergoing self-digestion and programmed cell death. Electron microscope studies of these cells show loss of mitochondrial inner membranes with ballooning and vacuolization of the mitochondria, indicating the first step in an irreversible cascade leading to programmed cell death.

MORE GLIOMA RESEARCH

Gliomas are cancers that originate in brain tissue. A 2004 report by Dr. Massi studied the effect of CBD on U87 and U373 human glioma cell lines. The beneficial effect of CBD appeared to be CB2 receptor-dependent and secondary to ROS generation (Massi et al., "Antitumor," 838). This is interesting because CBD normally does not interact with the cannabinoid receptors, but in some cases it clearly does. CBD caused a dramatic reduction in mitochondrial metabolism as measured by the MTT assay, resulting in an anti-proliferative effect and induction of apoptosis. This effect was partially blocked by addition of a CB2 receptor antagonist and by antioxidant Vitamin E (alpha-tocopherol). In a subsequent xenograft animal model, CBD injected into mice significantly inhibited the growth of implanted human brain cancer cells.

Another study by Dr. Massi elucidated the molecular pathways leading to apoptosis by CBD in a human glioma cell model (Massi et al., "The Non-Psychoactive," 2057). Dr. Massi demonstrated that mitochondrial release of cytochrome c, caspase activation, and ROS production triggered apoptosis in the CBD-treated human glioma cells. CBD-treated normal brain cells were left unharmed, again showing selectivity.

A 2013 report, again by Dr. Massi, treated human glioma cancer cells (U87-MG and T98G cells) with CBD. The results showed decreased cell proliferation and invasiveness in the treated cells (Solinas et al.) Examining protein expression, Dr. Massi found that the cancer cells pretreated with CBD showed a reduced amount of proteins involved in growth, invasion, and angiogenesis. CBD induced down-regulation of ERK and Akt signaling pathways in glioma cells. There was also decreased hypoxia-inducible factor HIF-1α in the treated cells. Dr. Massi showed that CBD's anti-cancer activity utilized multiple pathways. When one pathway is blocked or absent, another one is used to induce apoptosis.

PILOT STUDY IN NINE GLIOBLASTOMA PATIENTS

In 2006, Dr. Manuel Guzmán's group published its pilot study using THC infused directly into the brain tumors of nine patients with recurrent malignant glioblastoma (Guzmán et al., 197). The results of this pilot study were unimpressive. However, there may have been some benefit in two of the patients, and the THC was well tolerated and nontoxic. Brain biopsy material revealed the same molecular mechanisms in play as found in cell and animal studies. Specifically, cancer cells were induced to undergo programmed cell death, with evidence of both autophagy and apoptosis.

The lackluster results are actually not very surprising, and they bring up a very important point. Most people who have had success against cancer with cannabinoids have orally ingested much larger doses of whole-plant extract. There are no public testimonials of anyone injecting cannabinoids, and it is very likely no one has ever done it outside a lab setting. Oral ingestion allows cannabinoids to work systemically through the body, rather than locally, as with this experiment. Furthermore, whole-plant extracts benefit from the synergy of cannabinoids. The pilot study was still useful for showing that minor anti-cancer benefit was achieved and that THC was safe.

It is highly unfortunate that further clinical trials were not immediately started after this. In general, there is little interest from pharmaceutical companies in natural plant medicines they cannot patent, so there is much less funding for trials involving these medicines.

Breast Cancer, Id-1 Gene, and ERK/MAPK Signaling

Breast cancer is another type of aggressive cancer often with a poor prognosis. The study of this cancer led to the realization that CBD can influence genetics to inhibit a wide variety of cancers. Given the fundamental influence of genetics on health, this is a truly powerful anti-cancer mechanism.

CBD-INDUCED APOPTOSIS INDEPENDENT OF CANNABINOID RECEPTORS

CBD appears to cause programmed cell death in a manner independent of the CB1 and CB2 receptor system. As reported by Dr. Sean McAllister's group, the anti-cancer effect of CBD is at least partially related to down-regulation of the Id-1 gene through the ERK/MAPK pathway (McAllister et al., 37). Id-1 is a key regulator of cellular growth and cell cycle machinery involved in cell differentiation, maturation, senescence, and finally programmed cell death. Dr. McAllister's work demonstrated that CBD can actually work at the genetic level to inhibit cancers. While he has largely focused on breast cancer, the Id-1 gene is responsible for

116

promoting growth in other cancers as well, suggesting that CBD can inhibit multiple tumors through modifying genetics.

Dr. McAllister's group also reported that the combined use of THC with CBD has a synergistic effect with more profound suppression of cancer activity than the use of CBD alone (Marcu et al., 180).

Id-1 and Cancer Cell Biology

The Inhibitor of Differentiation (ID) gene is active in undifferentiated embryonal cells and generally inactive, or silenced, in well-differentiated, mature adult tissues. Many types of cancer have been found to possess highly active ID genes, which are thought to contribute to aggressive, metastatic, anaplastic behavior of these cell types. Increased Id-1 expression is associated with a more proliferative and aggressive cancer cell type. In addition, these cell types reverted to normal when the Id-1 gene was targeted and inhibited with antisense drug therapy. Therefore, the ability of CBD to down-regulate this gene is quite profound.

ERK/MAPK Signaling

The discovery of the ERK/MAPK signaling cascade (also known as the Ras-Raf-MEK-ERK pathway) was a major breakthrough in understanding cancer biology and has stimulated intensive efforts by the research community and pharmaceutical industry to develop inhibitors of ERK/MAPK signaling for cancer treatment (Roberts and Der, 3291).

The ERK pathway receives signals through receptors located on the outer cell membrane. These signals are then transferred to the cell nucleus to regulate gene expression. The ERK signaling cascade is involved in cell replication, growth, differentiation, and cell survival. Dysregulation of the ERK pathway leads to dysregulation of Id-1, which is a common occurrence in human cancers. Sean McAllister's group reports that CBD upregulates ERK signaling, which inhibits cancer cell proliferation and invasion via down-regulation of Id-1 genetic expression (McAllister et al., 38).

A testament to the versatility of CBD relates to how it kills brain cancer cells. One study found that CBD inhibited two kinds of glioma cells via down-regulating the ERK pathway (Solinas et al.). Depending on the type of cancer, CBD functions differently to inhibit it. This study is also examined further in a later section.

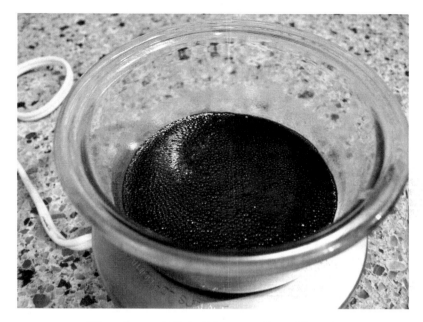

Filtered cannabidiol oil (courtesy Doug Flomer).

Mouse Models of Metastatic Cancer

In two mouse models of metastatic cancer, treatment with CBD significantly reduced primary tumor mass, size, and number of secondary lung metastases. Given that many other cancers share the Id-1 gene, it is likely these results would translate to other cancers as well. Dr. McAllister discussed this possibility in the conclusion of his group's paper.

The expression of Id-1 protein has been reported to be dysregulated in more than 20 types of cancer and suggested as a key determinant of tumorigenesis and/or metastasis in a wide range of tissues, including the breast. Reducing Id-1 expression (a gene whose expression is absent in most of the healthy adult tissues) could therefore provide a rational therapeutic strategy for the treatment of aggressive cancers (McAllister et al., 45).

SHRIVASTAVA'S GROUP AT HARVARD

Dr. Shrivastava's group at Harvard explored the molecular mechanisms by which CBD induced programmed cell death in breast cancer cells (Shrivastava et al., 1161). They examined CBD-induced apoptosis, autophagy, and generation of ROS in multiple human breast cancer cell lines. They found that CBD-induced cell death was concentration-dependent and applied equally to (ER+) estrogen receptor-positive and as well as (ER-) breast cancer cell lines. Furthermore, CBD preferentially killed cancer cells while having no deleterious effect on normal breast cells.

CBD's action was achieved independently of cannabinoid receptors. This suggested that the receptor mediating CBD in programmed cell death is yet to be discovered, at least in this case. Their model also demonstrated that within two hours of incubation of the breast cancer cells with CBD, there were signs of ER (endoplasmic reticulum) stress, which led to cell autophagy; in this case, autophagy was a prelude to complete programmed cell death. Dr. Shrivastava's further studies showed that apoptosis was associated with mitochondrial-mediated apoptosis through both intrinsic and extrinsic cell signaling pathways.

Leukemia

Early studies in 2003 by Dr. Gallily at Hebrew University in Jerusalem showed CBD-induced apoptosis via caspase activation in human leukemia cells (HL-60 cells). Giving the leukemia cells a short burst of radiation therapy prior to CBD enhanced the anti-cancer effect, attaining a 85–90 percent cell death rate. Normal white cells were left unharmed (Gallily et al., 1767).

Continuing Dr. Gallily's work, Dr. McKallip's group published in 2006 their studies of the effect of CBD on leukemia cells. They found CBD-induced apoptosis by activating CB2 receptors and increasing ROS (McKallip et al., 897). This is indeed fortuitous, because leukemia and lymphoma cell lines are known to over-express CB2 receptors. Other types of cancerous cells also have higher expression levels of cannabinoid receptors than their healthy counterparts, indicating that the body may be programmed to have cannabinoids induce apoptosis as a defense mechanism. If cancer cells are designed to express more cannabinoid receptors, they would be more susceptible to the apoptosis-inducing effects of cannabinoids.

Dr. McKallip acquired a patent in 2004 on the medicinal use of CB2 agonists, potentially including CBD, in lymphoma and leukemia. "The present invention relates to the targeting of CB2 cannabinoid receptors as a novel therapy to treat malignant lymphoblastic disease..." (Patent number U.S. 20040259936 A1).

Lung Cancer

Dr. Ramer's group at the University of Rostock in Germany published a 2012 report on CBD and lung cancer (Ramer et al., 1535). The study found early-onset upregulation (four-fold) of ICAM-1 (intercellular adhesion molecule–1) via cannabinoid receptors in CBD-treated lung cancer cells. At 48 hours later, they found upregulation of the tissue inhibitor of matrix metalloproteinases–1 (TIMP-1), which accounted for the loss of invasiveness of the lung cancer cells. The researchers also injected lung cancer cells (A549, H358, and H460) into mice and then treated them with CBD. The mice showed a two- to three-fold increase in ICAM-1 and TIMP-1 protein, which decreased cancer cell invasiveness. Upon microscopic inspection, the number of lung metastatic lesions had been reduced by half in the CBD-treated mice.

The increase in ICAM-1 also helps the body's own immune cells attach to and digest the cancer cells. Therefore, cannabinoids truly do work synergistically with the body to fight cancer.

Influences of Cannabinoids on Mitochondria and Metabolic Pathways

The effects of cannabinoids are diverse and multifaceted, working through many pathways to achieve both similar and different effects. Depending on what the body needs, cannabinoids seem to be able to adapt their function. The following are several ways by which cannabinoids affect many cancers through common mechanisms.

MITOCHONDRIA AND THE VOLTAGE-DEPENDENT ANION CHANNEL

Dr. Rimmerman from Tel Aviv University proposed another mechanism by which CBD triggers apoptosis (Rimmerman et al.). This mechanism involves the Voltage-Dependent Anion Channel (VDAC) at the outer mitochondrial membrane. It is a specialized membrane pore and a key regulator of mitochondrial function. Dr. Rimmerman showed that CBD acts directly on the VDAC to open the channel and increase membrane permeability. This allows the release of cytochrome c into the cytosol, which then activates the caspase proteolytic enzyme cascade and triggers programmed cell death in cancer cells. The exact receptors to achieve this have yet to be elucidated.

HEXOKINASE II: THE KEY TO CANCER

A key metabolic alteration of the cancer cell is the peculiar adoption of an embryonic enzyme called hexokinase II, which has an unusually high affinity for glucose and is attached to the VDAC on the outer mitochondrial membrane. If the enzyme could be detached, this would promptly trigger cancer cell death (Suh et al.). Perhaps targeting the VDAC membrane pore at the attachment of hexokinase II is the yet undiscovered mechanism of induction of programmed cell death by cannabinoids.

In a March 2013 paper, Dr. Suh lists 26 anti-cancer agents in Table I that target mitochondrial apoptotic signaling (Suh et al.). Included in this list is methyl jasmonate derived from the jasmine flower, a natural plant botanical. The anti-cancer mechanism of cannabis may be similar to that of methyl jasmonate. Studies by Dr. Cesari from Rio de Janeiro found anti-cancer activity of methyl jasmonate associated with detachment of hexokinase from the voltage-dependent anion channel, dissociating glycolytic and mitochondrial functions, decreasing the mitochondrial membrane potential, favoring cytochrome c release and ATP depletion, and activating pro-apoptotic and inactivating antiapoptotic proteins (Cesari et al.).

NUPR, THE SWISS KNIFE OF CANCER: STRESS-RELATED PROTEIN P8

Another possible mechanism for apoptosis is the p8 pathway. THC upregulates expression of the stress-regulated protein p8 (also known as NUPR1), a transcriptional regulator, which causes endoplasmic reticulum stress and may trigger programmed cell death via the intrinsic mitochondrial pathway or by autophagy (self-digestion of the cell, which often occurs before apoptosis). The NUPR1 gene has been dubbed the "Swiss Knife" of Cancer (Cano et al., 1439). The p8/NUPR1 pathway has been shown in glioma, pancreatic, and hepatic cancer cells. Dr. Manuel Guzmán speculates that perhaps this pathway may serve as the main mechanism by which cannabinoid receptor activation induces apoptosis.

CANNABIS AND THE P53 GENE

As discussed earlier, the p53 gene is a crucial regulator of apoptosis. Dr. Powles studied the effect of THC on leukemia cells, finding that apoptotic cell death occurred independently from the p53 gene pathway. This is a good thing, since the p53 pathway is inactivated in most cancer cells (Powles et al., 1214) Dr. Powles stated:

> One of the most intriguing findings was that THC-induced cell death was preceded by significant changes in the expression of genes involved in the mitogen-activated protein kinase (MAPK) signal transduction pathways. Both apoptosis and gene expression changes were altered independent of p53 and the Cannabinoid Receptors [Powles et al., 1214].

Selective for Cancer Cells— Leaving Normal Cells Unharmed

THC and CBD are the two major anti-cancer cannabinoids explored in research and used in practice by cancer patients. Unlike most chemotherapeutic agents, these cannabinoids selectively target cancer cells for apoptosis while sparing normal cells, which are left unaffected. While there has been progress in unraveling the molecular mechanisms of how cannabinoids induce programmed cell death in cancer cells, the mechanism for the sparing of normal cells has yet to be determined. Cancer cell selectivity is an obviously desirable feature. On the other hand, cytotoxic chemotherapy, the standard of care for cancer patients by mainstream oncology, has no selectivity and kills normal cells along with cancer cells. The lack of selectivity is responsible for the adverse side effects of chemotherapy, including nausea, vomiting, hair loss, chronic fatigue, anemia, and neuropathy.

Paola Massi, PhD, University of Milan

Paola Massi, PhD is a prolific cannabis researcher at University of Milan in the Department of Cellular and Molecular Pharmacology. Her

2013 article "Medical Cannabidiol—Is There Anything It Can't Do?" reviewed five different cancer types: breast cancer, glioma, leukemia, thyroid cancer, and colon cancer. She noted the type of cannabinoid receptor involvement, production of reactive oxygen species (ROS), molecular cell signaling, and presence or absence of autophagy and apoptosis in each of these cancers. Dr. Massi stated: "Cannabinoids possess anti-proliferative and pro-apoptotic effects and they are known to interfere with tumour neovascularization, cancer cell migration, adhesion, invasion and metastasization" (Massi et al., "Cannabidiol," 303).

DR. MASSI'S SUMMARIZING
STATEMENT ON CANNABIDIOL

Collectively, the non-psychoactive plant-derived cannabinoid CBD exhibits pro-apoptotic and anti-proliferative actions in different types of tumours and may also exert anti-migratory, anti-invasive, anti-metastatic, and perhaps anti-angiogenic properties. On the basis of these results, evidence is emerging to suggest that CBD is a potent inhibitor of both cancer growth and spread. The anticancer effect of this compound seems to be selective for cancer cells, at least in vitro, since it does not affect normal cell lines. The efficacy of CBD is linked to its ability to target multiple cellular pathways that control tumorigenesis through the modulation of different intracellular signalling depending on the cancer type considered [Massi et al., "Cannabidiol," 303].

Possible Pro-Cancer Effects of Cannabinoids

Some studies, or components of studies, have shown that isolated cannabinoids can actually increase the growth of cancer. These studies are by far dwarfed by anti-cancer studies, but their observations must be taken seriously.

A review study found that very low nanomolar concentrations of cannabinoids could cause epidermal growth factor-receptor and metalloproteinase-dependent cancer cell proliferation. However, when micromolar concentrations were used, cannabinoids induced apoptosis (Pacher, Bátkai, and Kunos, 450). Furthermore, whole-plant cannabis extracts have been shown to have even greater anti-cancer effect than isolated cannabinoids and at least in some cases do not have the pro-cancer effect when used at the lowest needed concentrations. One study found that in human DU-145 prostate cancer cells, the lowest doses of isolated plant cannabinoids tested had a stimulatory effect on cancer, but at the highest dose inhibition was observed. However, the CBD-rich whole-plant extract lacked the pro-proliferative effect even at the lowest concentration tested (Ligresti et al., 1380). Given that humans use whole-plant cannabis extracts in greater than micromolar concentrations, there is little danger of cannabinoids promoting cancer. The possibility of a pro-cancer effect in rare situations, however, should be a perpetual concern.

Corporate and Government Interest in Cannabinoids as Anti-Cancer Agents

While many natural substances show activity against cancer cells in cultures and animals, few are as potent as cannabinoids or attract as much attention. National governments and major corporations alike have shown strong interest in using cannabinoids to fight cancer in humans.

GW PATENT

In December 2013, GW Pharmaceuticals announced its patent (US 8790719 B2) for use of the cannabinoids THC and CBD in a 1:1 ratio for treating malignant gliomas ("GW Pharmaceuticals"). Sativex™ is their plant-derived cannabinoid prescription drug, which has a 1:1 ratio of THC to CBD. A clinical trial of Sativex in recurrent glioblastoma patients is currently under way and not yet completed.

MEDICINAL CANNABIS FDA-APPROVED FOR CANCER PATIENTS

Over the years, medicinal cannabis has traditionally been used to stimulate appetite and reduce nausea and vomiting of chemotherapy in cancer patients. Indeed, synthetic versions of THC, called Marinol® (dronabinol) and Cesamet® (nabilone), were both FDA-approved in 1985 for treatment of nausea and vomiting associated with cancer chemotherapy. In addition, cancer patients frequently suffer from pain as the cancer invades and destroys tissue. Both isolated cannabinoids and whole-plant extracts have been shown to be very effective in reducing the above symptoms and may actually be a better alternative to opiate pain pills. Opiates are addictive and cause a number of side effects like constipation that patients find unpleasant.

While these drugs are not necessarily intended to directly fight cancer, it is likely their ingestion still has some direct anti-cancer effect. Furthermore, patients who have less depression, nausea, and pain can tolerate traditional treatments better and thus have better outcomes.

ORPHAN DRUG STATUS

The United States has admitted that a cannabinoid could fight cancer in humans. In fall 2014, The U.S. Food and Drug Administration granted Insys Therapeutics orphan drug designation (ODD) for their CBD product "Insys" to treat gliomas. ODD is granted for drugs intended to treat conditions affecting less than 200,000 people. However, for a new drug to get this designation, there must be significant evidence that it could actually work. The fact that the FDA granted ODD to Insys indicates that they believe the evidence is strong enough to justify their approval.

Human Results

What matters foremost are the results of clinical trials with human subjects. Can cannabinoids actually fight cancer in humans? The testimony from many people from around the world strongly suggests that the answer is yes.

A CANCER TREATMENT IN YOUR BACKYARD GARDEN

In 2008, Rick Simpson, an early pioneer in the use of medicinal cannabis oil, released a documentary called *Run from the Cure*. In the video, he explains how anyone can make cannabis oil at home using simple equipment and raw cannabis buds. *Run from the Cure* also chronicled how Simpson grew cannabis in his garden, extracted the oil, and treated hundreds of people in his community. His experiences led him to believe that high–THC cannabis oil could effectively eliminate nearly any type of cancer and control nearly any type of disease.

At the time, he did not know anything about the endocannabinoid system or the myriad of studies, both past and yet to come, that would validate his observations. While many have improved upon his techniques and treatment methods since, there is no doubt he significantly raised awareness about the true potential of cannabis medicine and helped a lot of people.

Cannabis Oil Brain Tumor Remission

In a *Huffington Post* Interview, Dr. William Courtney discussed the case of an eight-month-old baby suffering from a malignant brain tumor ("Cannabis for"). The initial MRI scan showed typical features of an inoperable brain tumor, in this case a "butterfly glioma." This is characterized by invasion of the cancer into the corpus callosum, which divides the brain into left and right hemispheres.

The parents had declined conventional treatments like chemotherapy and radiation because of the risks. They decided to treat their child's brain tumor with cannabis oil instead. Miraculously, after two months of treatment with cannabis oil, the MRI scan showed dramatic improvement. Dr. Courtney remarked: "They were putting cannabinoid oil on the baby's pacifier twice a day, increasing the dose…. And within two months there was a dramatic reduction."

Follow-up scans indicated continued regression of the tumor. At four and at eight months, the scans showed more shrinkage, until it was virtually abolished. These results are highly significant given the nature of butterfly gliomas. They are highly aggressive and respond poorly to conventional treatments. The type of response seen in this case is almost never achieved. The incredible results are summed up in Dr. Courtney's statement, "The child is a miracle baby…. We should be insisting this is frontline therapy for all children before using medications that have horrific long-term side effects" ("Cannabis for").

Highly Aggressive Acute Lymphoblastic Leukemia in 14-Year-Old Girl

The following case report appeared in the November 2013 *Journal of Case Reports in Oncology* (Singh and Bali, 585). In March 2006, P.K., a 14-year-old girl suffering from weakness and spontaneous bleeding, was diagnosed with acute lymphoblastic leukemia (ALL), with more than 300,000 blast cells present on her peripheral blood smear. Her form of leukemia was highly aggressive with a positive Philadelphia Chromosome. P.K.'s leukemia was treated at the Hospital for Sick Children, Toronto, Canada with bone-marrow transplant, aggressive chemotherapy, and radiation therapy.

After 34 months, blast cells were again found in the blood; treatment was deemed a failure and further treatment futile. The doctors suspended all treatment and essentially gave up. The doctors noted in the chart: "The patient suffers from terminal malignant disease.... She has been treated to the limits of available therapy.... No further active intervention will be undertaken." The patient, P.K., was offered palliative treatment and sent home to die. While at home, the leukemia blast cell counts continued to increase, and frequent blood and platelet transfusions were required.

The family conducted their own research and found dramatic evidence of the anti-cancer potential of cannabis. Cannabis oil is generally well tolerated by chemotherapy patients to relieve nausea and vomiting, and the evidence showing potential against cancers themselves was enough for the family to further consider cannabis extract therapy.

Finding Rick Simpson and Phoenix Tears. The family found an organization known as Phoenix Tears, founded by Rick Simpson, from whom they learned how to prepare their own cannabis extract to be given orally to their daughter, P.K. With the introduction of this new cannabis oil treatment, the doctors observed a rapid dose-dependent reduction in leukemic blast cell count. This case is important because it shows in graphic form the potent anti-cancer effect of cannabis oil in acute lymphoblastic leukemia. Dr. Singh states: "The results shown here cannot be attributed to the phenomenon of 'spontaneous remission' because a dose response curve was achieved" (Singh and Bali, 591).

Although the treatment against the cancer itself was deemed a success, the patient ultimately succumbed to the toxic effects of chemotherapy. She died of a bowel perforation and peritonitis on day 78. A common side effect of chemotherapy, especially aggressive courses, is bowel perforations. This led the doctors to conclude the original treatment, not the cancer, was the cause of death, not the cancer.

What Is Evidence?

In spite of compelling basic science research, and inspiring case reports, mainstream medicine remains largely unconvinced. Without randomized controlled trials, traditional doctors will never accept cannabis extract medicine. It is true that a variety of trials, including double-blind randomized and open-label trials, are desperately needed to learn more about cannabis medicine. However, the scientific and existing anecdotal and clinical evidence clearly shows that cannabis extracts can combat many types of cancers. It makes no sense to make patients wait years for more trials when they have nothing to lose by using this treatment now. Increasing access would also increase data that could be collected from patients using the medicine. There is no doubt that trials will show that cannabinoids fight cancer; the question is how well do they work, what protocols optimize their effectiveness, and what are their limits.

Cannabis for Pain

Pain is a symptom of many diseases, and chronic pain is a condition in itself. For all of human history, people have experienced pain and sought ways to alleviate it. Pain is a necessary sensation; without it, we would not know something is wrong, and unnecessary deaths would dramatically increase. Unfortunately, when pain signals become uncontrolled, pain can be present even in the absence of real danger. Cannabinoids offer great promise for all types of pain, but especially chronic, neuropathic types for which opiate medications are almost completely ineffective.

A National Epidemic of Opiate Abuse

The convergence of politics with medicinal cannabis legalization is nowhere more evident than in mainstream medical treatment of chronic pain. Too many doctors are quick to prescribe opiate pain pills, leading to the narcotics abuse recognized by the Centers for Disease Control and Prevention (CDC) as a national epidemic (Sosin). Deaths from opiate pain pills have quadrupled since the early 1990s, when prescriptions skyrocketed as an outcome of drug marketing efforts.

While opiates are excellent medicines for acute pain, they are terrible for long-term chronic pain. Opiate narcotics are addictive, tolerance develops rapidly, and they can even lead to increased pain. Many people accidentally overdose and die using their legally prescribed medications. Unfortunately, modern medicine can do little for those with advanced pain, and the sickest among us are resigned to spend years barely managing their pain with high doses of opiates.

A SAFER ALTERNATIVE TO OPIATES FOR CHRONIC PAIN

In a 2011 report, Drs. Grinspoon and Aggarwal state: "Opioids may produce significant morbidity. Cannabis is a safer alternative with broad applicability for palliative care" (Carter et al., 297). There has never been a fatality from any use of cannabis. The reason for this is that unlike opiates, cannabis cannot cause respiratory depression, as there are virtually no cannabinoid receptors in the brainstem. Patients who overdose on opiate pain pills will fall asleep, stop breathing, and die. Patients who overdose on medicinal cannabis just fall asleep. Of course,

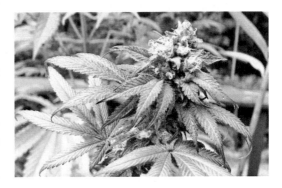

Cannabidiol-rich strains in ACDC, an indica/sativa hybrid (20 percent CBD and 1 percent THC (courtesy Doug Flomer).

there can be serious negative effects from a cannabis overdose, including severe anxiety and nausea. Through proper dosing and the use of cannabis medicines higher in CBD, these effects can be completely avoided.

A MORE EFFECTIVE ALTERNATIVE TO OPIATE PAIN PILLS

Medicinal cannabis allows chronic pain patients to decrease their doses and eventually wean off opiates (Abrams et al., 844). The medical evidence supporting the effective use of medicinal cannabis for pain control is now overwhelming (Ware et al., E694; Wilsey et al., 136; Fine and Rosenfeld; Ibrahim et al., 3093). A quote from Dr. David Baker writing in *Lancet Neurology* 2003 illustrates the profound effects of cannabinoids on pain.

> Cannabinoids inhibit pain in virtually every experimental pain paradigm either via CB1 or by a CB2-like activity in supraspinal, spinal, or peripheral regions, dependent on the type of nociceptive pathway being studied. This finding is consistent with high concentrations of CB1 receptors on primary afferent nociceptors, particularly in the dorsal spinal [Baker et al., 291].

An Unexpected Benefit:
Reduction in Mortality from Opiates

Reduction in deaths from opiate overdose was discovered as an unexpected benefit of medicinal cannabis legalization. In states where such laws have been implemented, doctors are free to replace opiate pain pills with safer and more effective cannabis preparations. This has resulted in a measurable decrease in patient mortality, as reported in a 2014 study from Dr. Marcus Bachhuber at Johns Hopkins Bloomberg School of Public Health. Public records from states that have legalized medicinal cannabis reveal a 25 percent lower mortality rate from opioid drug overdose compared to prohibitionist states (Bachhuber et al., 1668).

Neuropathic Pain

Neuropathic pain, which arises from nerves and often accompanies nervous system disorders, is usually treated with long-term opiate pain medications. This type of pain is especially resistant to traditional treatments, and even high doses of opiates have little effect. Cannabinoids offer great hope as a treatment for conditions involving neuropathic pain, including complex regional pain syndrome (CRPS) and fibromyalgia.

Medicinal Cannabis for Complex
Regional Pain Syndrome

Medicinal cannabis has been showing success against chronic refractory pain in CRPS. Dr. Mark Ware works at McGill University and presented his study of medicinal cannabis for complex pain at the 2010 annual World Congress on Pain in Montreal. His research indicated that an oral cannabinoid formula was "associated with up to 60 percent reductions in pain in 10 patients with refractory CRPS" (Wild). Furthermore, most of the patients were able to stop using their opiate medications and reported significant improvements in their quality of life.

Cannabis for Fibromyalgia Pain

Fibromyalgia is another pain syndrome with similarities to CRPS. It is very poorly controlled by traditional medicines. A survey of 1,300 fibromyalgia patients conducted by the National Pain Foundation and

National Pain Report found stunning results. It determined, "Medical marijuana is far more effective at treating symptoms of fibromyalgia than any of the three prescription drugs Cymbalta, Lyrica and Savella" (Anson, 2014).

For each of the FDA-approved drugs, at least 60 percent of respondents said the drug did not help at all. A maximum of 10 percent of respondents said the drug was very effective. The results were completely switched for medicinal cannabis. Only 5 percent of respondents said cannabis did not help at all, and 62 percent said it was very effective (Anson, 2014). Given that most of these people were probably smoking high–THC cannabis, one can only imagine the results if they used cannabis extracts with higher amounts of CBD.

STUDIES ON CANNABINOIDS FOR NEUROPATHIC PAIN

Dr. Elizabeth Rahn's 2009 review is an excellent summary of animal and human research on cannabis for neuropathic pain (Rahn and Hohmann, 713). Dr. Rahn reviewed the medical literature on cannabinoids for neuropathic pain associated with nerve injury, diabetes, chemotherapy-induced neuropathy, multiple sclerosis neuropathy, and herpes zoster neuropathy (shingles). She found that cannabinoids suppress neuropathic pain in nine different animal models of surgically induced traumatic nerve injury. She concluded that "clinical studies largely reaffirm that cannabinoids show efficacy in suppressing diverse neuropathic pain states in humans" (Rahn and Hohmann, 713).

DR. MARY LYNCH SYSTEMATIC REVIEW 2011

It is unusual for an off-patent generic drug or a natural substance to undergo randomized clinical trials in humans due to the associated expenses. Yet that is exactly what has happened for medicinal cannabis in pain management. For example, in 2011 Dr. Mary Lynch published a review of cannabinoids used for chronic non-cancer pain (Lynch and Campbell, 735). Dr. Lynch selected eighteen randomized trials "of excellent quality" from 2003 to 2010 evaluating cannabis for chronic pain, neuropathic pain, fibromyalgia, and rheumatoid arthritis. Fifteen of these eighteen trials (more than 83 percent) showed significant relief from pain compared with placebo. There was also improved sleep in the cannabis-treated group. Dr. Mary Lynch observed an anti-inflammatory effect as well and concluded that "cannabinoids are safe and modestly effective in neuropathic pain, with preliminary evidence of efficacy in fibromyalgia and rheumatoid arthritis" (Lynch and Campbell, 735).

Dr. Sunil Aggarwal Systematic Review 2013

In 2013, Dr. Sunil Aggarwal published an excellent summary of clinical trials of medicinal cannabis for allodynia, neuropathic pain, and other chronic pain syndromes (Aggarwal, 162). He found 38 published randomized trials; 27 (71 percent) of them concluded that cannabinoids are effective for pain-relief.

Mechanism of Action

Medicinal cannabis is effective for chronic pain because it reduces perception of pain, is anti-inflammatory, and affects voltage-gated sodium channels in nerves in similar ways as nerve blocking drugs such as lidocaine (Martin and Lichtman, 447; Nagarkatti et al., 1333). The voltage-gated sodium channels in nerves are thought to be important players involved with inflammation and neuropathic pain (Okura et al., 554).

Cannabinoids Induce Release of Endogenous Opioids

In an article published in 2005, researchers found that CB2 activation produced pain relief (antinociception) via the release of endogenous opioids (Ibrahim et al., 3093). This phenomenon explains the efficacy of medicinal cannabis for pain relief and also shows how exogenous opiates like Oxycontin can be reduced or eliminated. Heavy doses of pharmaceutical pain pills are no longer needed, as they are replaced by the body's own self-made opiates called endorphins.

Cannabinoids as Antioxidants and Neuroprotectants

In spite of the obvious rule that natural substances cannot be patented, the United States government has a patent on medicinal use of

"Cannabinoids as Antioxidants and Neuroprotectants" (US 6630507 B1). It would appear paradoxical that a government agency, The Department of Health and Human Services (HHS), would hold such a patent and at the same time another government agency, the Drug Enforcement Administration (DEA), would declare a ruling that cannabis "has no accepted medical use." Perhaps employees at the DEA should get up out of their chairs and walk across the hall to talk to the employees of HHS.

The antioxidant and neuroprotective properties of cannabinoids likely contribute to their analgesic effects.

Summary

The cell, animal, and human results are clear. Cannabis extracts have a role in the management of cancer and pain. Isolated cannabinoids and plant extracts have been shown to kill a wide variety of cancer cells through intrinsic metabolic pathways. THC exerts its effects predominantly by attaching to cannabinoid receptors and inducing apoptosis, whereas CBD largely uses non-cannabinoid receptor pathways, although in some cases it partially works through the CB2 receptor.

Clinical trials with humans are especially prevalent in pain-related conditions. The majority of these trials show that cannabis extracts are very effective against numerous forms of pain. Fibromyalgia in particular has no effective conventional treatment options, but medicinal cannabis has been reported to be the best treatment in self-reports from patients.

EIGHT

Research Studies
on Cannabidiol

The use of high-cannabidiol (CBD) cannabis extracts for treating medical conditions, especially epilepsy, has dramatically increased since the release of Dr. Sanjay Gupta's *Weed* documentary.

As a result, anecdotal reports have also exploded with stories of success, implicating CBD as an effective treatment in many types of epileptic conditions. While anecdotal data had been accruing for quite some time, the recent surge of both clinical trial and anecdotal reports in the press and on the internet has brought the benefits of CBD to the public's attention.

In addition to the rapidly growing evidence from regular individuals treating themselves and their children, the preclinical evidence supporting CBD's utility in treating a wide variety of conditions is very strong. Cellular and animal studies have shown that CBD has immense potential for treating almost any condition, including common and aggressive forms of cancer. However, there are relatively few large clinical studies documenting the use of CBD in humans, and most of the human results have accumulated outside an academic setting. This is because of CBD's novelty as a therapeutic compound and the federal restrictions imposed on research for any compounds derived from cannabis. Also, until recently, most cannabis strains had very low levels of CBD, so even those wishing to do experiments on CBD and other cannabis extracts were limited.

Thankfully, there are a few studies that have confirmed CBD's benefits in humans with seizure disorders, bolstering the notion that this phytochemical would work for other conditions as well. Once restrictions are removed and availability of CBD is increased, studies can flourish and

Opposite and 7 pages following: **Steps to make oil (courtesy Doug Flomer).**

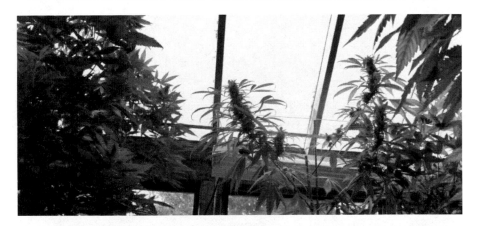

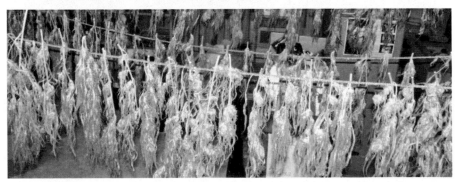

Top: **Very happy plants in an ideal greenhouse environment, everything grown organic, only medical grade Indica strains.** *Bottom:* **Hung out to dry! First harvest of Iranian Autoflower August 5, after 95 days' growth.**

further explore CBD's remarkable and wide-ranging benefits. Chapter Eight acquaints readers with the many medical applications of cannabidiol based on clinical trials, research studies, and anecdotal accounts.

Existing Scientific Studies

CBD is shown in preclinical models to potentially combat many disease conditions. However, the existing human studies examine CBD's effects only in a limited number of diseases, including multiple sclerosis, epilepsy, insomnia, social anxiety disorder, schizophrenia, bipolar disorder, Huntington's disease, cancer, and various kinds of pain (Zhornitsky and

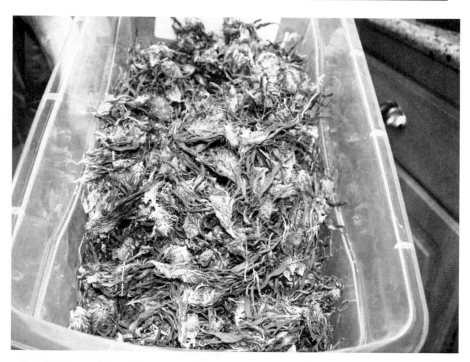

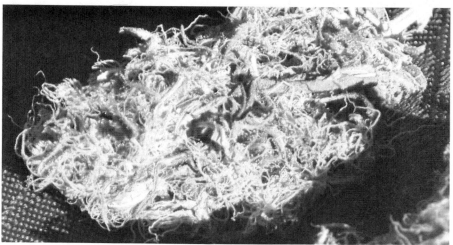

Top and bottom: Rough trim down to buds and sugar leaf. Heavy resin in buds.

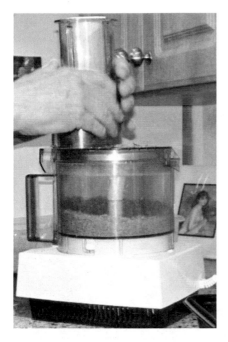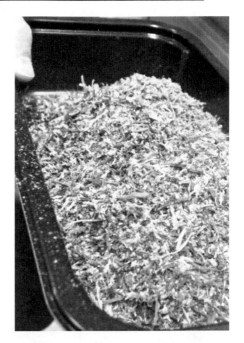

Buds ground and frozen before immersion in frozen alcohol. Freezing the alcohol results in more concentrated THC/CBD extract, less plant waxes and chlorophyll. The whole plant was not used, just the buds and bud sugar leaves.

Potvin, 529). The results clearly demonstrate the safety of CBD in humans, with varying levels of efficacy. While CBD does work on its own, the scientific and anecdotal data suggests it should be combined with other cannabinoids or terpenoids for maximum therapeutic effects.

The following studies primarily involve double-blind placebo-controlled models using human patients. In relevant situations, animal and cell studies are also explored, either because they shed light on the molecular mechanisms of CBD's therapeutic activity or they are the only studies available. Given how many cannabinoid-related cell-level results end up translating to humans, these studies are still quite indicative of the real-world potential of CBD.

Epilepsy

Chapter Six of this book explores how CBD combats seizure disorders, and some of the information on CBD in seizure disorders is summarized

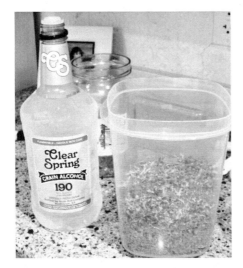

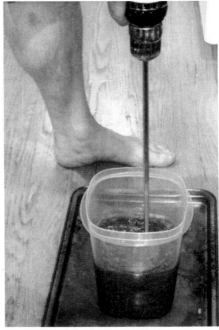

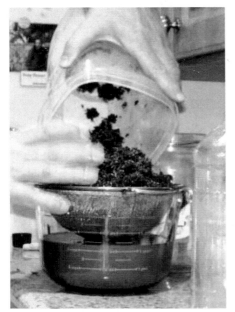

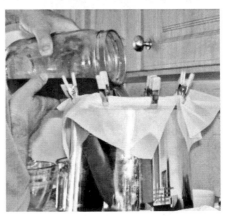

Agitated in food grade frozen alcohol, strained and filtered through silk screen into the distiller.

here as well. A 1980 study examining the use of CBD in healthy and epileptic patients found that the compound was well tolerated and produced no signs of toxicity (Cunha et al., 175). The study's double-blind, placebo-controlled experiment found that of eight patients in whom traditional medications failed to control seizures, four remained almost seizure-free and three improved partially during CBD administration. Only one did not improve at all, and in the placebo group, only one improved, indicating that CBD had a truly significant effect.

A 2013 study in *Epilepsy & Behavior* reported on nineteen parents using whole-plant high–CBD extracts for treating their epileptic children.

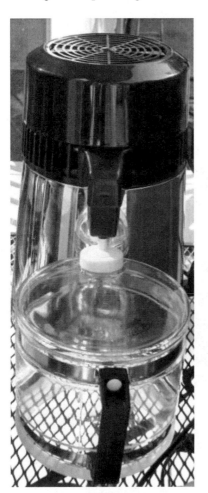

A standardized survey was used to measure the effectiveness of these extracts for several intractable forms of epilepsy. Thirteen children had Dravet syndrome, four had Doose syndrome, and the remaining two had either Lennox-Gastaut syndrome or idio-

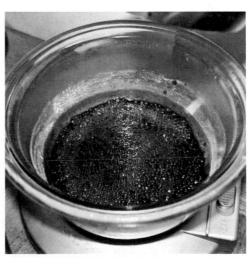

Distiller evaporates the Everclear, leaving the thick oil at the bottom of the distiller. Recaptures 50 percent of the alcohol. When mostly reduced, it is moved to coffee warmer for final reduction. If it bubbles more than the photograph above, it can overcook.

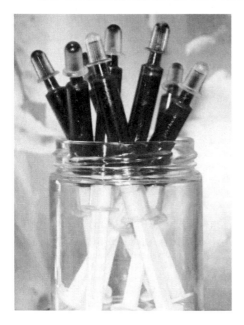

Final oil stored in 3 ml (or 3 gram) syringes. This is very strong cannabis oil. Further dilution in coconut oil may be necessary, but the concentrate is the best way to store it in the refrigerator. It is warmed to room temperature, or placed in a bowl of hot water to make it easier to push the syringe.

pathic epilepsy (Porter and Jacobson, 574). The majority of parents, sixteen, reported some kind of seizure reduction with the use of extracts. Six reported between 25 and 60 percent seizure reduction, eight reported a greater than 80 percent decrease, and two reported complete absence of seizures (Porter and Jacobson, 574). These parents had used an average of twelve pharmaceutical medications prior to trying cannabis oil, and these medications were completely ineffective at reducing seizures.

The supporting animal evidence is also quite strong. A 2012 study tested varying quantities of CBD on rodents using the acute pilocarbine model of temporal lobe seizure and the penicillin model of partial seizure (Jones et al., "Cannabidiol Exerts," 344). Amounts of 1, 10, and 100 mg/kg of CBD were used on both these models. In the former model, all doses were effective at reducing seizures. The same was true of the latter model, but the two higher dosage levels were more effective at significantly reducing the percentage mortality as a result of seizure. In a previous study, the authors had also determined CBD to be effective against a rodent model of pentylenetetrazole-induced generalized seizures (Jones et al., "Cannabidiol Displays," 569). That study also used two *in vitro* models of epilepsy, finding that CBD decreased various physiological measures of epileptic activity. These effects were mediated by CB1-receptor independent mechanisms that have yet to be fully explored.

GW PHARMACEUTICALS TRIALS

The UK-based company GW Pharmaceuticals has been exploring the use of isolated cannabinoids and cannabis extracts to treat cancer,

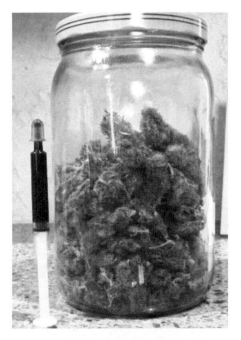

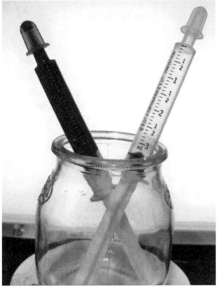

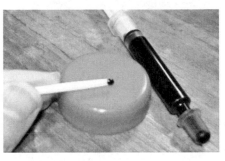

Undiluted cannabis oil is VERY strong.

3 ml syringe = 1 ounce of cannabis bud.

Each 3 ml tube is the reduced oil from 1 oz. of buds.

Each 1 ml tube is the extracted oil from 9 grams of buds, about 9 joints.

It is diluted with coconut oil for topical application, to make the oil easier to spread.

All doses should be tested first at the smallest amount, and increased gradually each night until desired effects.

Dose administered under the tongue can take 15–60 minutes to take effect.

epilepsy, multiple sclerosis, and pain. Their most well known and used product is Sativex, which is a 50/50 mix of THC and CBD. Several of the studies mentioned above used this medication as the source of cannabinoids. Sativex is approved for use in the UK and in more than 20 other countries including Canada, but it has not yet been approved for use in the United States (Gardner).

In response to the growing interest in CBD, GW researchers have also developed a new product called Epidiolex. This product is delivered via a syringe dropper, rather than being sprayed under the tongue like Sativex. It consists of 98 percent CBD, zero THC, and small quantities of other cannabinoids (Gardner, "Doctors Stress"). Epidiolex was developed to combat rare forms of epilepsy, and GW had already funded research establishing the safety and efficacy of CBD as an anti-seizure and anti-inflammatory agent. In December 2013, the U.S. Food and Drug Administration approved Phase II clinical trials of Epidiolex. Epidiolex comes in a viscous liquid form, in doses of 25 mg/meter or 100 mg/meter to be dispensed from syringes. The FDA gave approval for two intermediate-sized clinical trials sponsored by two doctors, Dr. Orrin Devinsky, a professor in the Department of Neurology, Neuroscience and Psychiatry in the New York University School of Medicine and director of the NYU Comprehensive Epilepsy Center; and Dr. Roberta Cilio, a pediatric neurologist at the University of California, San Francisco,

GW Pharmaceuticals released physician-collected information in June 2014. Results were from 27 patients, nine of whom had Dravet syndrome. For all patients, the average reduction in seizure frequency over 12 weeks was 44 percent, with 15 percent of patients seizure-free at the end of the period ("GWPharma"). The results were more profound for the Dravet patients. Their frequency was 52 percent, and 33 percent of patients became seizure-free. These improvements are very promising given the novelty of Epidiolex and the relatively short treatment period.

Social Anxiety

Nearly everyone experiences some form of social anxiety at some point in their lives, but for a small portion of the population, this anxiety is substantially detrimental to normal functioning. A double-blind study in *Neuropsychopharmacology* with 24 social anxiety disorder (SAD) patients examined the effects of 600 mg of CBD on anxiety during public speaking. This dose "significantly reduced anxiety, cognitive impairment, and discomfort in their speech performance" (Bergamaschi et al., 1219). The placebo group did not experience these benefits.

Another study determined that 400 mg of CBD could reduce anxiety in SAD patients (Crippa et al., 121). Relative to placebo, this dose significantly reduced subjective anxiety, as determined by functional neuroimaging. The anxiolytic effects were ascribed to activity in the limbic system of the brain.

PAIN CONDITIONS

The use of cannabis for the side effects of chemotherapy and the pain associated with cancer is well known. A 2004 double-blind, placebo-controlled study tracking patients using THC, CBD, or THC:CBD extracts over 12 weeks found they were effective at providing symptomatic control, with the extracts having THC proving most efficacious (Notcutt et al., 440). Different patients required a range of dosing protocols for optimal relief, indicating the individualized nature of cannabis treatments. The observed side effects were generally acceptable.

Another 2004 double-blind study found both THC:CBD and THC extracts reduced pain and improved sleep in patients with brachial plexus avulsion, a spinal cord condition resulting from injury (Berman, Symonds, and Birch, 299). While the pain levels did not fall by the rate predicted in the hypothesis, the medicine was well tolerated, with most adverse events resolving spontaneously.

A 2010 study found that a THC:CBD extract was effective at relieving treatment-resistant cancer pain. A THC extract reportedly lowered pain as well, but the results were not statistically significant. Compared to placebo, twice as many patients using the THC:CBD extract experienced a 30 percent reduction in the utilized pain scale (Johnson et al., 167). Some adverse effects were noted, including mild to moderate increases in nausea and vomiting, but overall the extract was effective for the majority of patients.

SCHIZOPHRENIA

Most people associate cannabis with causing schizophrenia. This is because of media reports of studies suggesting that THC can precipitate the condition in people who are already predisposed to it. However, these studies only demonstrate correlation, and there is no evidence that proves that cannabis or THC can actually cause schizophrenia. It is very likely that people with the condition attempt to use cannabis as a way to self-medicate.

However, given the psychoactive nature of THC and its ability to cause some negative mental effects, such as anxiety and paranoia, there is certainly the chance that it could be problematic for some patients. Strains that are higher in CBD or other non-psychoactive cannabinoids are probably better suited for individuals with schizophrenia or other mental disorders.

A double-blind study that compared CBD to amisulpride, a potent antipsychotic, showed that the cannabinoid was about as effective as the traditional option (Leweke et al.). Patients were administered 800 mg of CBD per day for four weeks. The study found that CBD was even more effective than amisulpride when it came to alleviating the negative symptoms of schizophrenia, such as absence of motivation or emotional responses. As importantly, CBD had very few side effects, making it a markedly superior choice.

In a *Time* article about the study, co-author Dr. Daniele Piomelli stated, "The results were amazing. Not only was [CBD] as effective as standard antipsychotics, but it was also essentially free of the typical side effects seen with antipsychotic drugs" (Szalavitz). Such side effects include potentially permanent movement disorders like tardive dyskinesia and weight gain. Disorders of this type were seen in the amisulpride group but not the CBD group.

On a functional level, it was determined that CBD's antipsychotic effect was achieved via inhibition of the degradation of anandamide, the body's chief endocannabinoid. This also suggests that schizophrenia may arise from an endocannabinoid deficiency that phytocannabinoid supplementation can correct.

Another study used 29 patients with first-episode onset schizophrenia, as described in a review by Dr. Antonio Waldo Zuardi (Zuardi et al., "A Critical Review," 5132). This double-blind study compared CBD with placebo, finding that 18 patients experienced a significant reduction in psychotic symptoms as compared to baseline. It was also notable that while 10 people dropped out of the placebo group, only one did so in the treatment group.

One study using only a few patients did not show much efficacy. A 2010 study in the *Journal of Psychopharmacology* examined three patients using CBD monotherapy for treatment-resistant schizophrenia (Zuardi et al., "Cannabidiol Monotherapy," 683). One patient improved mildly while the two others showed no improvement. However, there were no side effects and the treatment was very well tolerated.

In a later summarizing study by Dr. Zuardi, the author explained that the two non-responding patients had especially severe, refractory cases of schizophrenia that did not even respond to clozapine (Zuardi et al., "Cannabidiol, a Cannabis," 423). He cited the double-blind CBD vs. amisulpride study as an example where the cannabinoid was very effective. He also described a patient case study involving a 19-year-old schizophrenic female who significantly improved during treatment but experienced worsening symptoms when treatment was interrupted (Zuardi et al., "Cannabidiol, a Cannabis," 425). Again, a lack of side effects supported the immense safety profile of CBD.

GENERAL ANTIPSYCHOTIC
POTENTIAL AND SAFETY

For more than 30 years, there has been continuously growing evidence that CBD may possess certain antipsychotic properties. Dr. Zuardi's extensive review of this evidence, which included analyzing the safety of CBD, was published in 2012 (Zuardi et al., "A Critical Review," 5131). The first study to suggest antipsychotic effects appeared in 1982 and found that people using THC and CBD together had less anxiety and psychosis-like symptoms than people using THC alone. CBD does not lower THC levels in the blood but exerts its mitigating effects by antagonizing the CB1 receptor.

Subsequent animal studies showed that CBD had immense potential as a medicine, with a chemical profile similar to conventional atypical antipsychotic drugs. It is also useful at low doses for helping with social withdrawal. Unlike these drugs, CBD is virtually devoid of side effects even at higher-than-needed doses (Zuardi et al., "A Critical Review," 5134).

The *in vitro* and *in vivo* animal studies suggested that CBD was non-toxic and would not cause any side effects, serious or minor. When CBD was administered acutely through various routes of administration to healthy volunteers, no toxic effects were observed (Zuardi et al., "A Critical Review," 5135). Chronic administration of a wide range of doses also elicited no negative effects. One study examined healthy people using between 10 and 400 mg of CBD per day, and another analyzed volunteers using as much as the exorbitantly high dose of 1,500 mg per day. Even at the highest doses, there were no behavioral side effects. However, because CBD and THC are metabolized through the cytochrome P450 pathway in the liver, high doses can inhibit the metabolism of other drugs. When combining cannabinoids with traditional pharmaceuticals, it is best to take them at different times so that they are both absorbed properly.

The 1982 study mentioned above was the first of several endeavors to ascertain the effects of co-administered cannabinoids. Several studies between 2000 and 2010 found that CBD reduced positive psychotic symptoms from THC administration and reduced impairment (Zuardi et al.,

"A Critical Review," 5136). A 2008 study examined long-term cannabis users by analyzing the presence of cannabinoids in hair. Subjects with only THC showed higher levels of positive psychotic symptoms, whereas those with THC and CBD or no cannabinoids in hair had fewer symptoms.

CBD also appears to counter the memory impairment notoriously associated with cannabis consumption. A 2010 study with 134 cannabis users found those using high–CBD varieties had no memory impairment, whereas those using low–CBD varieties had marked impairment (Zuardi et al., "A Critical Review," 5136).

CBD can also attenuate the psychotic effects of other non-cannabinoid substances. A randomized study administered ketamine along with CBD or placebo to ten healthy volunteers. Those receiving CBD had better psychomotor activation, which is generally inhibited by ketamine use, as well as reduced depersonalization symptoms (Zuardi et al., "A Critical Review," 5136). As ketamine symptoms often mimic those found in schizophrenia, this study also suggested that CBD could treat schizophrenia. The cannabinoid may be effective for non-life-threatening overdoses of ketamine or other psychedelic drugs, as such overdoses can be very unpleasant or mentally challenging for users.

Given this evidence, it is quite possible that chronic use of high–THC cannabis could precipitate schizophrenia or other psychotic disorders in populations predisposed to it. However, the original, wild species of cannabis had much higher levels of CBD until breeders began cultivating strains to be higher in THC. As breeders begin to reintroduce CBD back into the marketplace and more people learn of its benefits, the problems observed with chronic high–THC cannabis use will hopefully dissipate.

Dr. Zuardi's summarizing study concluded by mentioning CBD's similarity to traditional antipsychotics, but without the side effects. It also stated the important need for new antipsychotic drugs. Given CBD's proven usefulness in animal studies and its remarkable safety, more studies are warranted. At this point, anyone wishing to try CBD as a potential replacement for current antipsychotic medications should be allowed to do so.

Parkinson's Disease

Given the proven neuroprotective properties of cannabinoids, it makes sense that they would therapeutically benefit Parkinson's Disease

(PD), which is neurodegenerative in nature. Progressive loss of dopamine producing neurons in the basal ganglia is the defining feature of this chronic neurodegenerative disease. Medical science can only speculate as to the cause of progressive loss of dopamine producing neurons in the basal ganglia, a defining feature of Parkinson's Disease. Common symptons include tremor, slowed movement (bradykinesia), muscle stiffness, balance, posture and speech problems. Thankfully, cannabinoids show great promise in the treatment of Parkinson's Disease.

In general, cannabinoids have been shown to hold promise in the treatment of all major central nervous system disorders, including traumatic brain injuries and stroke. They are very effective at inhibiting the excitatory neurotransmitter glutamate, which is toxic when it activates receptors too frequently and in high concentrations (Croxford, 2003). The inhibition of reactive oxygen species and the inflammatory tumor necrosis factor also plays a role.

An animal study using a rat model of PD illuminated a key mechanism by which CBD exerts its neuroprotective properties. When administered directly after dopaminergic cell death, CBD was able to recover the dopamine depletion (García-Arencibia et al., 162). However, when administered one week after the event, the compound was not effective. CBD's neuroprotective effect was purportedly derived from upregulation of superoxide dismutase, one of the body's key and most powerful internal antioxidants. These effects were mediated partially by the CB2 receptor, receptor-independent effects, and possibly influences from other receptors. Another study found that a high–CBD cannabis extract was effective at protecting neurons in a key area of the brain associated with PD (García et al., 1495). THCV was found to have neuroprotective properties as well, which were at least partially mediated by the CB2 receptor and antioxidant effects.

A symptom which sometimes arises in PD patients is rapid-eye-movement sleep behavior disorder (RBD). It is characterized by the loss of muscle atonia during sleep and thus active movement during dreaming. A 2014 study examined the effect of CBD on four patients with RBD stemming from PD. All four patients experienced a "prompt and substantial reduction" in how many RBD-related events they experienced (Chagas et al., "Cannabidiol Can Improve," 564). The patients did not experience any side effects, pointing to remarkable tolerability and efficacy.

A double-blind study followed 21 PD patients using placebo, CBD 75 mg per day, or CBD 300 mg per day (Chagas et al., "Effects of Cannabidiol," 1088). It was conducted by the same team as above in the same year. It found the 300 mg level of CBD was effective at improving well-being and quality of life for the patients but did not exert motor benefits or possible neuroprotective effects. More trials were recommended with larger samples and more specific objectives.

Schizophrenia and PD share a common feature in that they involve disruptions in dopamine levels. With schizophrenia and other forms of psychosis, there is thought to be a hyperactive dopamine state, whereas in Parkinson's there is a dopamine deficiency. Interestingly, CBD can positively affect psychosis in both cases. A 2009 study, again by Dr. Zuardi, evaluated six patients who used CBD for four weeks in various doses, starting at 150 mg per day (Zuardi et al., "Cannabidiol for the Treatment," 979). The patients continued using their other medications. While on the CBD treatment, there was a significant decrease in symptoms as measured by two psychiatric scales. CBD also generally improved symptoms according to the Unified Parkinson's Disease Rating Scale.

MULTIPLE SCLEROSIS

Like PD, multiple sclerosis (MS) has received considerable attention as a therapeutic target for cannabinoid medicines. It is a neurodegenerative disorder characterized by loss of the myelin sheath on nerve cells. This fatty layer helps facilitate neural messages and protect the cell. In MS, the immune system attacks the myelin sheath, thus impeding cellular communication and increasing the susceptibility of neurons to death.

A 2003 study tested THC, CBD, and a 1:1 THC:CBD extract against pain, spasticity, and bladder control issues in 24 patients, 18 of whom had MS. Both THC and CBD were found to provide significant pain relief, as well as improve bladder control, muscle spasms, and general spasticity (Wade et al., 21). The researchers concluded that cannabis extracts can improve neurogenic symptoms unresponsive to standard treatments. The minor side effects that did occur were predictable and well tolerated. With further treatment, it is likely that such effects would become increasingly manageable.

A study one year later in *Multiple Sclerosis*, which used relatively similar parameters, found that both THC:CBD and THC whole-plant extracts were effective in normalizing bladder function in 15 evaluated patients (Brady et al., 425). On average, urine urgency, number and volume of incontinence episodes, and nocturia were significantly reduced after treatment. In addition, patients reported improvement in pain, spasticity, and quality of sleep measures. There were few serious side effects.

ALZHEIMER'S DISEASE

As people begin to grow older, more are being diagnosed with some form of dementia. One in three seniors dies with dementia. The most well known form is Alzheimer's disease (AD), which affects more than five million people in the United States and is the sixth leading cause of death ("Latest Facts"). There are few effective treatments, and it is virtually impossible to reverse the trajectory of dementia when it begins. For most people, their best hope is slowing it down.

Unfortunately, there are no existing human trials that have explored the effects of CBD on any form of dementia. However, promising evidence from cell and animal studies suggests that the compound would be very beneficial. Anecdotal evidence from doctors and caregivers who have worked with dementia patients suggests that cannabis extracts in general are remarkably effective for even the most severe cases.

AD is thought to result from the build-up of beta amyloid protein, which leads to plaque that interferes with neuronal signaling. The beta amyloid accumulation also causes neuroinflammation, which leads to excitoxicity and neuronal cell death. Intracellular tangles formed by hyper-phosphorylated tau protein also contribute to the disease and may even be the main cause.

CBD has been shown to directly reduce beta amyloid production by interacting with amyloid precursor protein (Scuderi, Steardo, and Esposito, 1007). The addition of CBD modifies this protein, reducing full-length protein levels. Most importantly, this results in an increased survival of neuronal cells. Neuroprotection is critical to delaying or reversing the onset of AD. Although CBD does not interact strongly with CB1 or CB2 receptors, it has been shown to directly activate the peroxisome proliferator-activated receptor-gamma. Through the activation of this special receptor, CBD confers at least some of its neuroprotective effects.

A study by Dr. Giuseppe Esposito confirmed that CBD positively influenced beta amyloid-induced neurotoxicity via PPAR-gamma (Esposito et al., "Cannabidiol Reduces"). It also showed that CBD could stimulate neurogenesis, the growth of new neurons, in the hippocampal region of the brain. Given that the symptoms of AD ultimately result from the death of neurons, being able to replace these cells is critical to total healing.

The mechanisms of CBD's neuroprotective effects are varied and powerful. A study exposed cells to beta amyloid protein and found it reduced cell survival by increasing reactive oxygen species, lipid peroxidation, caspase–3 (pro-apoptotic enzyme) activation, DNA fragmentation, and increased intracellular calcium (Iuvone et al. 134). CBD treatment prior to the beta amyloid exposure decreased all five of these measures, leading to significantly elevated cell survival. Interestingly enough, when CBD is exposed to cancerous cells, it induces programmed cell death by increasing several of these exact same measures, demonstrating the remarkable ability of cannabinoids to distinguish between healthy and damaged cells.

Although there have not been any human studies, the fact that CBD's abilities extend to animals is very promising. A 2007 study by Dr. Esposito injected mice with beta amyloid protein, which caused increases in a variety of neuroinflammatory responses (Esposito et al., "Cannabidiol in Vivo," 1272). CBD administration was found to inhibit the expression of all measured neuroinflammatory markers, leading the authors to conclude that this was a promising pharmacological tool for fighting this type of inflammation.

One of the most recent studies yielded profound results when testing CBD on a mouse model of AD. Chronic CBD treatment was able to reverse cognitive deficits related to social recognition and novel object recognition (Cheng et al., 3009). In an interview with the *Sydney Morning Herald*, one of the study's authors, Dr. Tim Karl, remarked on the effectiveness of the treatment. "It basically brings the performance of the animals back to the level of healthy animals. You could say it cured them, but we will have to go back and look at their brains to be sure" (Corderoy).

ANTIBACTERIAL EFFECTS

Methicillin-resistant Staphylococcus aureus (MRSA) bacteria are serious threats to individuals who become infected. These unique types of bacteria cannot be treated effectively with current antibiotics. MRSA has become increasingly more prominent as antibiotic use has increased, as the unnecessary use of such medicines creates more resistant strains.

Cannabinoids represent a unique approach to this issue. A study previously described in Chapter Five found that CBD and four other cannabinoids had potent activity against several MRSA strains (Appendino). However, the antibacterial effects of CBD and THC have been known since as early as 1976, when a study showed that relatively low concentrations of the compounds could kill staphylococci and streptococci bacterial cells (Van Klingeren and Ten Ham, 9).

CARDIOVASCULAR DISEASES

Heart disease is the leading cause of death in the United States, followed by cancer. Cannabinoids are quickly proving to be, based on the scientific and anecdotal evidence, effective treatments for both of these top killers. CBD in particular has a wide range of therapeutic benefits for several cardiovascular issues.

While there are no clinical trials examining the effects of CBD on cardiovascular performance in humans, the preclinical evidence is extremely promising and suggests that CBD would be beneficial for many issues.

Restricted blood flow is the primary cause of damage to the cardiovascular system, as cells begin to die when they do not receive adequate amounts of oxygen and glucose. A 2010 study explored the effects of CBD administered to mice before coronary ischemia was induced (Walsh et al., 1234). The CBD-treated mice had a reduced number of arrhythmias (irregular heartbeats) and infarct size (volume of tissue death resulting from loss of oxygen). Reperfusion injury was also shown to be susceptible to CBD. Although it seems counterintuitive, the restoration of blood flow after it has been cut off can induce further damage. In this case, CBD also reduced infarct size. The study concluded that CBD was cardioprotective in the acute phase of ischemia and reperfusion.

A previous study in 2007 that specifically focused on reperfusion injury found that CBD-treated animals experienced a 66 percent reduction in infarct size compared to the control animals (Durst et al., H3602). This improvement was associated with a reduction in inflammatory markers. Too much inflammation is a key process behind much of the damage associated with cardiovascular diseases, so reducing inflammation is an effective cardioprotective mechanism.

People living with diabetes often suffer from heart conditions stemming from their primary diagnosis. Several characteristics of diabetes-related heart problems extend to other cardiovascular conditions as well. A study in the *Journal of the American College of Cardiology* illustrated the remarkable benefits of CBD, as shown through separate mouse and human cell studies. A wide variety of inflammatory and fibrosis biochemical markers were significantly reduced via CBD treatment (Rajesh et al., 2115). General myocardial dysfunction was also attenuated. Perhaps most importantly, oxidative and nitrative stress was reduced, leading to increased survival of heart muscle cells. The study also examined how CBD affected human cardiomyocytes that were exposed to high levels of glucose. Such levels significantly increase reactive oxygen species generation, which can lead to cell death. As with the mouse observations, CBD inhibited these dangerous oxidants and protected cells from death (Rajesh et al., 2115).

High glucose levels can also lead to the development of atherosclerosis, which is a hardening of the arteries. Fat, cholesterol, and white blood cells accumulate in the walls of arteries to form plaque. This is why the anti-inflammatory benefits of CBD are so important, because they help prevent this accumulation. A 2012 study found that CBD, through its immunomodulating properties, could reduce the progression of atherosclerosis induced by high glucose levels (Kleiner and Ditrói, 499).

A 2013 study summarized the extraordinary potential of CBD as a treatment for cardiovascular diseases. By examining the bulk of relevant scientific literature, the study's authors concluded that CBD could protect against several types of vascular damage through varied antioxidant and anti-inflammatory-based effects (Stanley, Hind, and O'Sullivan, 313). It also suggested further work, and thus clinical trials, of CBD in humans to explore whether these effects would translate. The existing anecdotal evidence strongly suggests that when trials are carried out, they will be positive.

Gastrointestinal Diseases

Many people suffer from some type of gastrointestinal disease. Forms of inflammatory bowel disease, which include Crohn's disease and ulcerative colitis, are especially detrimental to patients. Given that anti-inflammatory effects are among the chief benefits of cannabinoids, it makes sense that these diseases would respond to cannabis treatments.

A 2013 study carried out in Israel found that even smoked cannabis was effective at drastically mitigating or even eliminating Crohn's disease. Although the study used a high–THC form of cannabis, there were small amounts of CBD present, and the authors suggested a larger follow-up study with nonsmoked cannabis, likely including forms with higher levels of CBD (Naftali et al., 1276).

The double-blind, placebo-controlled experiment included twenty-one patients with severe forms of Crohn's disease who did not respond to traditional therapy, including steroids and immunomodulators. Patients in the treatment group smoked cannabis cigarettes containing 115 mg of THC twice daily. A very significant clinical response was seen in ten of eleven subjects, with five achieving full remission (Naftali et al., 1276). Only one person in the placebo group achieved remission, and only four achieved a response. Three cannabis patients were able to wean themselves from steroid dependency. All patients using cannabis reported improved sleep and appetite, with no significant side effects.

Dr. Jeffrey Hergenrather, the president of the Society of Cannabis Clinicians, reported in *O'Shaugnessy's* on his work with 38 patients, 28 with Crohn's disease and 10 with ulcerative colitis ("Hergenrather Presents"). On average, the results were very remarkable—pain reduced by half, stools per day reduced by a third, vomiting was reduced, and appetite increased. Most importantly, the patients' overall quality of life increased significantly. Half of the patients were able to stop their daily use of pharmaceuticals, although many did require those medicines for "flare-up" periods. The article emphasized, "Hergenrather's results strongly suggest that herbal cannabis is beneficial in the treatment of irritable bowel disorders" ("Hergenrather Presents").

Cell and animal studies strongly support these human-level results. Researchers in a 2009 study induced colitis in mice, then treated them with CBD (Borrelli et al., 1111). The compound reduced colon injury and several inflammatory markers, leading the researchers to conclude that CBD could prevent experimental colitis in mice. They also used human adenocarcinoma cells to measure CBD's effect on oxidative stress, as reducing such stress is a potential mechanism of gastrocytoprotective actions. After administration, reactive oxygen species production and lipid peroxidation were reduced. A 2011 study that used cultured human-derived colonic biopsies found that CBD counteracted the inflammatory environment (De Filippis, et al.). These anti-inflammatory effects were also seen in mice that had externally-induced inflammation, as reflected by reductions in inflammatory markers.

DIABETES

Type I and Type II diabetes affect millions of people throughout the world and involve the body's inability to correctly process glucose. While there has been relatively little research into cannabinoids and diabetes, the existing evidence is quite promising, especially since there are few treatments for diabetes besides insulin supplementation.

A 2006 study tested CBD on non-obese diabetes-prone mice, which are highly susceptible to the autoimmune disorder Type I diabetes. CBD treatment reduced the incidence of diabetes from 86 percent in control mice to 30 percent in treated mice (Weiss et al., "Cannabidiol Lowers," 143). The researchers, including Dr. Raphael Mechoulam and Dr. Lola Weiss, also examined the pancreases of these mice, finding that CBD reduced inflammation of the islets of Langerhans, where insulin is made. Direct tissue destruction by autoantibodies and cytokine-induced inflammation are the direct causes of Type I diabetes; therefore, CBD may be effective for either prevention or even treatment of this disease.

Another study in 2008 by the same team used mice that were in a latent diabetes stage or had initial symptoms of diabetes (Weiss et al., "Cannabidiol Arrests," 244). In this case, diabetes was diagnosed in 32 percent of the CBD-treated group, whereas 100 percent of the control group developed the disease. Pro-inflammatory and anti-inflammatory markers were decreased and increased respectively, pointing to the mechanisms of CBD's protective effects. As with the previous study, examination of pancreases revealed more intact islets, demonstrating that CBD prevented their destruction.

Implications of Studies

All natural cannabinoids are currently listed as Schedule I substances in the United States Controlled Substances Act, indicating that they have no medical use. The above studies, and many others not discussed here, clearly indicate that cannabinoids have incredibly potent medical applications. This has been demonstrated through very precise cell and animal studies and, more importantly, in a number of double-blind, placebo-controlled studies.

Therefore, the first implication of these studies is that cannabis must be immediately removed from Schedule I. Doing so would allow natural cannabinoid products to be prescribed in the right settings. Doctors are currently permitted only to "recommend" cannabis in states where it is legal, and this does not even include the right to advise patients on how best to use the medicine (although that is starting to change). Modifying the law will allow physicians to maximize the use of medicinal cannabis, while not affecting the state of recreational cannabis matters.

The second implication is that far more research is needed. The scientific community has collectively learned much about which conditions cannabinoids can benefit, but so many mechanisms of action remain elusive. Moreover, many studies have been limited to cells and animals, whereas human studies are most needed. Once the legal environment is changed, clinical trials will be far easier. Also, as institutions become more educated on the profound benefits of cannabis medicine, funding from private entities and governments, including state authorities and perhaps even the federal government, will certainly increase.

Summary

Cannabidiol has been shown to benefit sufferers from practically all major diseases. In cases where there are no controlled clinical trials, there is promising cell and animal-based evidence that suggests that the compound would benefit humans. Given that many cannabis trials have confirmed that preclinical results do translate to humans, it is likely that human trials of CBD for diseases with previous positive animal studies of effectiveness with CBD would also show positive results.

The mechanism of action of CBD is generally unrelated to the traditional cannabinoid receptors, including CB1 and CB2. Other receptors, including peroxisome proliferator-activated receptor-gamma, are targets for CBD. Working through this receptor and receptor-independent pathways, CBD exerts antioxidant, anti-inflammatory, and anti-apoptotic effects to protect healthy cells from foreign and autoimmune threats. These general mechanisms enable CBD to combat an extensive variety of diseases, and as more research is conducted, its utility will probably only grow.

NINE

Legal Issues, Cannabis Farming and Politics

In his book *The Cult of Pharmacology*, Richard DeGrandpre explains that because drugs occupy a socially animated realm, it is difficult, if not impossible, to know how much of what is observed as a drug effect is due to the drug as a pharmacological agent and how much is due to the drug as an object to which a whole set of beliefs, rituals, and expectations have been attached (17). Cannabis is the perfect example of a drug in which expectations of its abuse potential, rather than unequivocal proof, have led to laws, incarcerations, seizures of property, and restrictions on medical research.

As we learned in earlier chapters, unlike opiates and benzodiazepines, cannabis is not by definition an addictive substance. Because receptors for cannabis are sparse in the brain stem, cannabis doesn't affect the cardiovascular system or respiration. For this reason, cannabis has never caused a fatal overdose. Like any substance, including water, untoward physiological effects can occur when too much cannabis is consumed, particularly in edible products with high THC content. Nevertheless, hysteria fostered by fears of cannabis being addictive and toxic, along with aggressive anti-cannabis lobbying by competing industries, incited political decisions in 1969 that led to the current status of cannabis as a Schedule I drug. Chapter Nine focuses on the legal and political history of cannabis and its current legal status.

Patent vs. Ethical Drugs

At the turn of the twentieth century, the most significant drugs consumed included alcohol, opiates, cocaine, and marijuana. By mid-century, alcohol remained as the only one of these substances that hadn't fallen from grace. Even during the alcohol prohibition years, physicians commonly wrote prescriptions for the use of alcohol as medical therapies, and alcohol was available at speakeasies.

By the end of Prohibition, when concerns over alcohol abuse receded, cannabis's uses as a medical therapy came under question. The reasons were not related to the effectiveness of cannabis. They were related to yellow journalism and textile companies opposed to the competition from hemp fiber. Little attention was paid to the many ancient and current medical uses of cannabis.

As a therapy, cannabis was first introduced in Europe and the United States as a patent tonic or elixir. Pharmaceutical companies, which began flourishing in the 1930s with the advent of synthetic prescription drugs, cooperated with the American Medical Association (AMA) to recommend safe, "ethical" prescription drugs over patent medicines. It was financially advantageous to both the pharmaceutical companies and physicians to promote the notion that patent medicines were inferior.

In order to legitimize drug use under the guise of medical treatment, stimulants as well as sedatives were widely prescribed to treat the stresses of everyday life. Advertisements in medical journals described amphetamines as the perfect tonic for depression and barbiturates as a necessary aid for sleep. The burgeoning business of prescription medications as a panacea for every ailment imaginable was considered legitimate and ethical as opposed to patent medicines, which were inexpensive. By the early 1940s, cannabis patent medicines had become highly taxed, rarely prescribed, and, consequently, removed from the U.S. Dispensary.

Racial Issues, War Protestors and Pot Smokers

However, cannabis remained popular among jazz musicians, academics, artists, and students. An allegiance to cannabis was viewed by law enforcement agents as an act of disobedience and rebellion against authority. This perception also contributed to cannabis's status as an illegal drug when compared to legitimate, ethical pharmaceuticals. In 1930 New Orleans, marijuana was blamed for the first refusals of black entertainers to wear blackface and for black musicians playing lively music that incited foot-tapping (Herer, 123). Journalists reported that Mexicans under the influence of cannabis were asking that their children be educated and making other insolent demands.

In the 1950s through the late '60s, cannabis use was widespread on American campuses. When student groups began protesting the Vietnam War, the general opinion of law enforcement agents was that the students' views were a result of cannabis intoxication.

Federal Opposition

In September, 1969, then President Richard Nixon initiated Operation Intercept, an attempt to reduce the influx of Mexican marijuana and to get Mexico to crack down on Mexico's cannabis farmers. Eventually, Mexico complied and burned a few marijuana fields. U.S. Deputy Attorney General Richard Kleindienst explained that "since marijuana is not addictive," students wouldn't resort to crime to get it (Lee, *Smoke*, 117). His remark that marijuana is not addictive contradicted the basic tenets of the Federal Bureau of Narcotics, which had recently been re-christened the Bureau of Narcotics and Dangerous Drugs (BNDD). Kleindienst, however, had done his homework and knew that there were no studies or any proof that cannabis was addictive. On the contrary, studies indicated that cannabis was not an addictive substance.

A complete failure, Operation Intercept did cause the price of cannabis to rise. Consequently, the drug became more attractive to Americans. While Mexico remained a major source of marijuana in the 1970s, Americans began traveling to the Near East, Afghanistan, India, and Nepal and returning with smuggled bricks of hash. The Brotherhood of Eternal Love, an underground network of surfers and bikers, smuggled Afghani hashish into the U.S, which they processed into oil and distributed throughout North America, making a fortune along the way.

The Controlled Substance Act

In preparation for passing the Controlled Substance Act (CSA), enacted as Title II of the Comprehensive Drug Abuse Prevention and Control Act of 1970, Nixon personally chose members who shared his own anti-drug stance to form a committee known as the Shafer Commission to study and document the marijuana problem. When Nixon realized that the committee was not finding a problem with marijuana, he advised Shafer to change his tune and made mention of a potential appointment to a federal judgeship (Lee, *Smoke*, 121).

Undeterred, Shafer and his team released its report, "Marihuana: A Signal of Misunderstanding," in March 1972. The title sums it up. At 1,184 pages, the report estimated that 24 million Americans had smoked marijuana at least once and that there were no differences between users and non-users. The commission found no inherent problems with cannabis but saw it as a "symbol of the rejection of cherished values" because its public use was something of a protest by young adults. The committee went on to say that there was an extensive degree of misinformation about marijuana and there was no need for politicizing the marijuana issue. They found that no evidence that marijuana caused physical or psychological problems and that it did not lead to the use of hard drugs. Furthermore, there was no evidence of even one human fatality resulting from marijuana intoxication. In summary, they felt that the potential harm of getting arrested was worse than any problem caused by cannabis itself. In this report, the Shafer Commission called the application of the criminal law in cases of personal use of cannabis "constitutionally suspect," and declared that "total prohibition is functionally inappropriate" (Sacco and Finlea, 4).

Rejecting its policy recommendations, Nixon never read the entire report but went on to sign the Controlled Substance Act of 1970, which officially classified marijuana, along with heroin and LSD, as a Schedule I drug with no medical benefits. The Schedule I categorization was listed as a caveat in which the classification was supposed to be temporary and reevaluated by a special federal commission (Fox, 54). When the Shafer Report was published, the recommendation to reclassify marijuana was ignored, although more than 30 states passed bills that reduced penalties for possession.

In addition to the strange schedule drug classifications that were introduced, the Controlled Substance Act eliminated mandatory minimum drug sentences. Nevertheless, Congress reinstated them in the 1980s. Regardless of what medical experts and advisory committees thought, the U.S. Justice Department passed The Controlled Substance Act, and Governor Shafer was never appointed to the federal bench (Lee, *Smoke*, 23). Since 1970, despite numerous recommendations by medical researchers, physicians and activists to reclassify cannabis, the government has ignored a series of federal reports and recommendations and refused to comply.

Decriminalization Efforts

Efforts to decriminalize marijuana continued to fail through the next decade. In August 1977, President Jimmy Carter told Congress he supported ending all federal penalties for marijuana possession up to one ounce. Despite his recommendation, research into the medical properties of cannabis was curtailed, and the DEA, which replaced the BNDD, became more vigorous in its efforts to seize marijuana and personal property and to destroy cannabis plants, fields, and farms.

The National Academy of Science Report

In 1981, the National Academy of Sciences (NAS) prepared a report stating that the federal classification of cannabis as a Schedule I drug with no medical value was false and harmful to efforts to decrease drug use. President Reagan never acknowledged or publicized the NAS report. The similar findings of the LaGuardia Commission, the Shafer Report, and the NAS report were pushed to the back burner, where they've since remained.

Presidents Ronald Reagan and George H.W. Bush kept up the charade of the War on Drugs, and President Bill Clinton steered clear of the issue. Having financial ties to Pfizer, Eli Lilly, and other drug companies, Bush actively lobbied illegally both within and without the administration as vice president in 1981 to permit the dumping of unwanted, obsolete, or especially domestically banned substances on unsuspecting Third World countries (Herer, 65). In addition, Bush appealed to the Internal Revenue Service for special breaks for certain drug companies manufacturing in Puerto Rico. In 1982, Vice President Bush was ordered to stop lobbying the IRS on behalf of drug companies by the U.S. Supreme Court (Herer, 65). Richard DeGrandpre, a past fellow of the National Institute on Drug Abuse (NIDA), summarizes the situation in writing, "No doubt the war on drugs will one day rank among the most shameful periods in American history" (174).

The DEA and Turbulent Times

The War on Drugs has been costly for both the United States and its residents. As a result, millions of Americans have wasted years in jail, lost their jobs, and had their property seized by the series of events that Anslinger and yellow journalists set into motion. As recently as 2001, in

Vandalia, Michigan, DEA agents and local law enforcement agents killed cannabis advocates Tom Crosslin and Rollie Rohm, who had protested efforts to have their property, Rainbow Farm, seized under forfeiture proceedings (Kuiper, 22).

By 1993, hundreds of thousands had been victimized by civil asset forfeiture. Under civil forfeiture, all one's possessions can be seized without indictment, trial, or conviction. Suspicion of offenses has been enough to justify seizure of cars, home, bank accounts, and businesses. On May 6, 1992, a well known physician, Jonathan Wright MD, stood by as heavily armed agents of the FDA raided his office and held his employees at gunpoint while they confiscated laboratory equipment, patient records, computers, and reference books. The reason for the raid was to seize Dr. Wright's supply of B vitamins and L-Tryptophan, harmless nutritional supplements. No arrests were made and the FDA dropped the case four years later (Wollstein).

In 2010, the DEA eliminated approximately 10.3 million cultivated pot plants (this number excludes feral hemp plants, tens of millions of plants typically seized and destroyed annually by the DEA). By 2011, the total number of seized plants fell to 3.9 million, largely as a result of reduced plant seizures in California. This is largely due to the downsizing of, and then ultimately the disbanding of, the state's nearly 30-year-old Campaign Against Marijuana Planting (CAMP) program. In 2012, DEA-assisted marijuana seizures in California had fallen 73 percent since 2010—from a near-record 7.4 million cultivated pot plants eradicated in 2010 to approximately 2 million in 2012. However, DEA-assisted cannabis eradication efforts have remained basically the same in other leading grow states during this same period.

While plant seizures continue to be on the decline, property seizures have increased. According to the DEA's 2012 statistical report (Drug Enforcement Agency), the total number of cannabis plants eradicated nationwide fell 42 percent between 2011 and 2012 and continues on a downward trend. In 1989, the asset value of forfeitures amounted to $285,000,039, with amounts steadily climbing, the last report from 2010 showing a forfeiture asset value amount of $1,786,567,692 ("Asset Forfeiture").

Judge Examines Legality of Schedule I Classification

In May 2014, Judge Kimberly J. Mueller in California made headlines when she challenged the classification of cannabis as a schedule I drug.

The case centered around six men charged with growing cannabis on national forest land on October 3, 2011. Mueller's decision was based on a footnote written by U.S. Supreme Court Justice John Stevens in 2005 regarding the medical efficacy of cannabis. At the hearing in November 2014, medical experts validated the medical uses of cannabis, and former drug czar Bertha Madras stated that the potential for addiction in cannabis was too great, although she could produce no studies to back her claims. The final ruling is expected in 2015 (Haglage).

Advocacy Groups and Legal Groups

Advocates for changing the Schedule I classification of cannabis, such as the National Organization for the Reform of Marijuana Laws (NORML) and world-renowned researchers such as Raphael Mechoulam, have stated that research conducted worldwide through 1976 suggests that if cannabis were legal, it would immediately replace 10–20 percent of all pharmaceutical prescription medications (Herer, 66). It's not surprising that opposition to the reclassification of cannabis comes primarily from the pharmaceutical industry. By definition, Schedule I drugs have no medical use and cannot be used safely even with a doctor's supervision. By 1970, when cannabis was appointed to Schedule I classification, medical uses of cannabis were well known. In 1972, NORML petitioned for the transfer of cannabis to Schedule II so that it could be legally prescribed. Since then, other groups including the Drug Policy Foundation and the Physicians' Association for AIDS Care have joined forces with NORML.

Hearings conducted before the Bureau of Narcotics and Dangerous Drug (BNDD) were especially instructive. As Lester Grinspoon writes in his book on the history of cannabis, he witnessed a proposal to classify the synthetic opiate analgesic pentazocine (Talwin) as a Schedule I drug. Despite testimony detailing hundred of cases of addiction, several fatal overdoses, and evidence of abuse, pentazocine was made a Schedule IV drug with minimal restrictions. And incredibly, at these same hearings, the petition to reclassify cannabis was rejected on the grounds that this would violate U.S. Treaty obligations under the United Nations Single Convention on Narcotic Substances (Grinspoon and Bakalar, 14). The BNDD also, violating the law, refused to have an additional public hearing. In January 1974, NORML filed suit against the BNDD.

In 1975, the DEA, successor to the BNDD, acknowledged that treaty obligations would not be violated by a reclassification but refused to conduct further public hearings. In 1980, the Second Circuit Court of Appeals reversed the BNDD's dismissal of the petition, remanded the case for reconsideration, and criticized the BNDD as well as the Department of Justice.

Although the synthetic form of THC, drobinol, was classified as a Schedule II drug in 1985, cannabis and natural THC failed efforts to be reclassified during two-year hearings lasting until 1988, despite recommendations by the ruling administrative law judge, Francis Young, that cannabis should be reclassified to Schedule II (Grinspoon and Bakalar, 15). Despite the failure of the DEA to follow Judge Young's recommendations, the views of Judge Francis Young are commonly cited in successful Medical Necessity Defense petitions, such as those of glaucoma patients Robert Randall and Elvy Musikka (Zeese, 22–3).

Groups supporting reclassification of cannabis included the nonprofit Alliance for Cannabis Therapeutics; the Cannabis Corporation of America, a pharmaceutical firm interested in extracting natural cannabinoids as therapies once cannabis was moved to Schedule II; and the Ethiopian Zion Coptic Church, which supported the use of cannabis in religious rituals. Opposing groups included the DEA; the International Chiefs of Police; and the National Federation of Parents for Drug-Free Youth (Grinspoon and Bakalar, 15). This is especially interesting considering how many parents of children with seizure disorders are now among the largest supporters for reclassification and how many law enforcement officers are in favor.

Even though Judge Young said that approval by a significant minority of physicians documenting that cannabis had medical applications was enough to challenge the Schedule I classification, the DEA disregarded his opinion. The plaintiffs appealed, only to face a final rejection of all pleas in March 1992.

Hemp Products

In a 2001 press release, the DEA announced rules to clarify the status of hemp products ("DEA Clarifies Status"). Because THC is found in all parts of the cannabis plant, including hemp, federal law prohibits the use of any products from which THC may enter the human body, such as energy drinks or snack bars, made from hemp and containing THC. However, if products such as soaps, lotions, shampoos, clothing, birdseed products, rope, twine, and cosmetics do not contain THC that can be ingested, they can be imported into the United States.

States vs. Federal Government

The efforts of patients such as Robert Randall to obtain cannabis for his severe glaucoma led to rare instances where the federal government begrudgingly provided limited amounts of medical cannabis to patients. However, these patients remained at risk of the government's sudden refusal to comply. To dispense cannabis, state agencies first had to receive FDA approval for an Investigational New Drug (IND) application for either individuals or groups. The IND program allowed for patients who had exhausted all other treatments to obtain potentially curative drugs not yet FDA approved for marketing. The IND program included a provision in which physicians were required to describe a lengthy, specific research protocol for each patient. From inception in 1976 until 1992, after which no new patients were admitted, the IND program provided limited amounts of cannabis to patients via the National Institute on Drug Abuse (NIDA). As of 2014, four patients are still receiving medical cannabis under the IND program ("U.S. Federal Farm").

This process soon became a nightmare, with only ten states, including New Mexico, eventually establishing programs for the medical use of cannabis. Understanding that government resources couldn't be counted on, in 1978, New Mexico enacted the first medical marijuana law for patients with glaucoma and chemotherapy-related nausea. A young cancer patient, Lynn Pierson, is largely credited for the success of New Mexico's programs, although, due to interference by the FDA, she died before ever benefitting from the use of cannabis. Thirty-five states followed New Mexico by 1992, but the states soon found their own laws difficult to implement.

While the state programs were never able to run in the way they were intended, they did show that cannabis, and to a lesser extent THC, were able to relieve symptoms of nausea, glaucoma, and appetite loss related to AIDS. However, interference from federal agencies led to persecution by federal authorities, including seizure of plants and criminal charges. Today, while the federal government appears to be tolerant of state programs, the state programs are always under the threat of government intervention. As of December 2014, 23 states and the District of Columbia have successfully implemented medical marijuana programs.

Measures to Legalize Cannabidiol

With cannabidiol frequently spotlighted in the daily news, state lawmakers who have steadfastly opposed legalizing cannabis are now singing the praises of cannabidiol. While these well-meaning gestures show a measure of compassion, lawmakers need a greater understanding of the cannabis plant and the ways in which the individual components, including the psychoactive cannabinoid THC, work together (see Chapter One). There's a misconception that THC is bad and CBD good, with little understanding of the health benefits and pharmacokinetics of these compounds. A greater pool of controlled clinical studies documenting the efficacy of either the whole plant and/or THC exists (Armentano, 1). States with laws allowing for limited access to low–THC, high–CBD strains include: Alabama, Florida, Iowa, Kentucky, Mississippi, Missouri, North Carolina, South Carolina, Tennessee, Utah and Wisconsin ("State Medical Marijuana").

The Research Ban

After the identification of delta–9–tetrahydrocannabinol (THC) by Mechoulam in 1964, a number of research studies indicated a tremendous therapeutic potential for cannabis. Overall, these studies confirmed the medical benefits of cannabis that were described more than 5,000 years ago. This was a terrifying prospect for pharmaceutical companies.

Consequently, the formal research ban on cannabis instituted in 1976 was the result of American pharmaceutical companies successfully petitioning the federal government to be allowed to finance and evaluate 100 percent of medical research. In 1976, the Ford administration, NIDA, and the DEA proclaimed that no American independent research or federal health program would be allowed to again investigate natural cannabis derivatives as medicines. Pharmaceutical companies were allowed to investigate THC but could not conduct research on any of the other potentially therapeutic cannabis compounds, including more than 400 other cannabinoids, terpenoids, and other plant phytochemicals.

The Status of Cannabis Research

The federal government makes no bones about being opposed to cannabis research focusing on medical benefits. However, research geared toward trying to prove negative effects of cannabis abounds. On its website, the Office of National Drug Control Policy explains, "The Administration steadfastly opposes legalization of marijuana and other drugs because legalization would increase the availability and use of illicit drugs, and pose significant health and safety risks to all Americans, particularly young people" ("Marijuana Fact Sheet"). This statement is particularly disconcerting considering the number of children with seizure disorders, such as Lydia Shaeffer (Taylor), who died in the past several years before she could obtain cannabidiol oil.

The federal government vigilantly guards university research related to cannabis with an iron fist. Necessary funding from the National Institutes of Health (NIH) is limited and under constant scrutiny. Even when funding is approved, cannabis extracts are not always available. Little interest is paid to impressive trial results, especially when they show the superior benefits of cannabis compared to those of pharmaceutical agents.

NIH Funding for Medical Cannabis Research

A review conducted in January 2014 showed that while most of the research conducted by NIDA involves drug abuse, the NIH funded 28 trials involving the medical benefits of cannabis and cannabinoids (National Institutes of Health). Medical conditions under investigation for benefits from cannabis and cannabinoids include autoimmune diseases, inflammation, pain, psychiatric disorders, seizures, and substance use disorders (SUDs).

The National Institutes of Health also reported that from 1999 through June 2014, only 16 studies using government farm-produced cannabis that did not request NIH funding have been approved. For approval, researchers must have their projects cleared through a Department of Health and Human Services (HHS) scientific review panel. They must also obtain an approved IND application from the Food and Drug Administration (for human studies) as well as a Drug Enforcement Administration registration for a Schedule I controlled substance (for all studies.)

The United States Government Cannabis Farm

The only NIDA-sponsored cannabis farm, the Marijuana Research Project, is located at the University of Mississippi and is operated by a team of nine. In 2013, the National Institute on Drug Abuse paid the university $847,000 to run the facility, which provides cannabis for approved researchers across the country.

According to Mahmoud Elsohly, PhD, Director of the NIDA Marijuana Project, for decades the farm has only produced strains high in THC with no or negligible CBD.

But with heightened interest in CBD and other cannabinoid extracts, Dr. Elsohly and his team are hoping to offer new strains. According to Dr. Elsohly, in early 2014 his team successfully cultivated a second variety of marijuana containing equal amounts of CBD and THC. Later in 2014, he hopes to grow a high–CBD, low–THC variety similar to strains used for seizure disorders ("U.S. Federal Marijuana Farm").

Sue Sisley and Research into Cannabis for PTSD

In 2014, the psychiatrist Sue Sisley found her research into cannabis for post-traumatic stress disorder (PTSD) at the University College of Medicine halted by the federal government. Sisley first received approval for her research from the Food and Drug Administration in 2011 while working at the Department of Veteran Affairs. Because the study involved cannabis, two additional levels of approval were required. Permission from the DEA is necessary to possess and transport the drug, and approval is needed from the National Institute on Drug Abuse (NIDA) to carry on the research. If the research has not received funding from the NIH, additional approval from the HHS is needed. In an article in the *Washington Post*, Orrin Devinsky, director of the epilepsy center at New York University's Langone Medical Center, stated that many would-be cannabis researchers are driven to abandon their projects after discovering how expensive and time-consuming it can be to obtain cannabis for their research (Cha, Ariana, 3).

Fired for Lack of Funding

The University of Arizona fired Sisley on June 27, 2014, stating that funding for her project, a project that took four years to get off the ground and showed that cannabis offers considerable promise in PTSD, was running out and that the telemedicine program she worked with was shifting direction (Galvan, 1). In an interview with CNN, Sisley said that the university didn't like the optics of veterans smoking and vaporizing marijuana on their campus even in an FDA-controlled trial. Similar to other reports, a literature review of U.S. National Library of Medicine files showed that of 2,000 studies on marijuana, only 6 percent investigated medical benefits (Young, "Medical marijuana research").

Funded by the State of Colorado

In November 2014, Sue Sisley received a $2 million grant from the state of Colorado to continue her research of cannabis's effects on veterans with PTSD. Sisley reported that she will now be able to conduct her research without relying on an Arizona University laboratory. Her study, which she will conduct through her private practice, will be split between participating veterans in Arizona and at Johns Hopkins University in Baltimore.

On December 17, 2014, Colorado reported awarding more than $8 million for medical marijuana research in response to complaints that little is known about cannabis's medical potential (Wyatt B1). The grants were awarded by the Colorado Board of Health and will go toward studies on cannabis in epilepsy, brain tumors, pain (in comparison with oxycodone), irritable bowel syndrome, Parkinson's disease, and two studies on post-traumatic stress disorder. Some of the studies are still awaiting federal approval (Wyatt, B3). In recent years, California has been the only other state to earmark state funding for clinical cannabis research.

Agriculture Laws

On February 7, 2014, President Obama signed the Farm Bill of 2013 into law. Section 7606 of the act, Legitimacy of Industrial Hemp Research, defines industrial hemp as distinct and authorizes institutions of higher education, or state departments of agriculture in states where hemp is legal, to grow hemp for research or agricultural pilot programs. Industrial hemp is defined in the Farm Bill as any part of the Cannabis sativa L plant, whether growing or not, which contains no more than 0.3 percent THC on a dry-weight basis.

States with laws making industrial hemp legal include California, Colorado, Hawaii, Indiana, Kentucky, Maine, Montana, Nebraska, North Dakota, Oregon, Utah, Vermont, Washington, and West Virginia. The states are able to establish their own regulations regarding industrial hemp research and pilot programs. Farmers interested in growing hemp must be certified by their state's department of agriculture and they must be conducting research or starting an approved pilot program. Sales and marketing of hemp are allowed under these provisions ("2014 Farm Bill").

Practical Applications

Amid the newly formed hemp industry in Colorado, in December 2014, Colorado's Stanley Brothers, the developers of Charlotte's Web, announced plans to greatly expand by the summer of 2015. Besides producing industrial hemp in their massive new facility in Uruguay, the opportunity to grow industrial hemp in Colorado will allow them to supply their cannabidiol-rich oil to 3,500 people in Colorado and California by the end of January 2015 (Rodgers, Jakob, A1).

Congress Passes Medical Marijuana Protection Bill

In December 2014, Congress passed a federal spending bill that contains protective measures for state medical marijuana and industrial hemp programs. The spending bill includes an amendment that prohibits the Department of Justice from using funds to go after state-legal medical cannabis programs. If the bill is signed into law, the federal government will stop its raids on medical marijuana dispensaries.

The bill protects medical marijuana programs in the 23 states that have legalized marijuana for medical purposes, as well as the 11 additional states that have legalized cannabidiol oils. Under the Obama administration, the DEA and several U.S. attorneys have raided marijuana dispensaries and sent people to prison even though they complied with state laws. According to a report released last year by advocacy group Americans for Safe Access, the Obama administration has spent nearly $80 million each year cracking down on medical marijuana, which amounts to more than $200,000 per day (Ferner).

Summary

Although the medical benefits of cannabis have been confirmed for centuries, political decisions implemented in the 1930s have led to laws that ultimately led to a ban on the medical uses of cannabis. With the classification of cannabis as a Schedule I drug in 1970, medical research has been curtailed, and individuals growing or obtaining cannabis for medical conditions have been prosecuted and had property seized.

With research in the last decade confirming the benefits of cannabis extracts in seizure disorders, cancer, multiple sclerosis, and other conditions, state laws have been passed allowing for the medical use of cannabis in 23 states and the District of Columbia. A number of other states have approved the medical use of cannabidiol extracts. New laws regulating hemp farming are making medical cannabis extracts high in cannabidiol more available, although government regulations on cannabis research and funding remain stringent and cannabis remains a Schedule I drug.

TEN

Notable Individuals in the Cannabis Extract Movement

The rising use and legitimacy of medicinal cannabis is a truly unique phenomenon in history. Unlike other medical revolutions, this one has not been led by doctors. Due to the placement of cannabis as a Schedule I drug with no medicinal use, conventional physicians are banned from formally prescribing cannabis to their patients. Even in states where medicinal use is legal, doctors are limited to "recommending" cannabis under their free speech rights. They still cannot actually prescribe cannabis and, to the detriment of patients, usually cannot provide advice about how best to use cannabis medicine.

The legal environment has turned dispensary owners and caregivers into doctors. Since licensed physicians are normally not allowed to say anything beyond, "Cannabis might help you," other channels are the only ways for patients to gain information. Thankfully, some doctors in certain situations are starting to give more instruction, but this is not the standard. By integrating knowledge from caregivers, online sources, and existing scientific studies, patients can make more informed decisions and optimally use cannabis. This chapter describes some of the major players who are bringing cannabis extracts to the forefront.

Inherent Problems

Restricted access is one of the two great problems the legal prohibitions created. This alone has led to the suffering and even deaths of thousands of people who otherwise might have been saved with cannabis extracts. The limits on research have been perhaps equally as damaging.

The Schedule I placement of cannabis has made it extremely difficult for researchers to study the plant's phytochemicals and their medicinal properties. Research proposals have to be approved by numerous government agencies, and these agencies are reluctant to support research into the medicinal use of cannabis, although studies that aim to discredit cannabis are well funded.

Dr. Donald Abrams, an oncologist discussed later in this chapter, remarked on the many challenges in conducting federally approved research. When he spoke with the National Institute on Drug Abuse (NIDA) about such research, it stated, "We're the National Institute on Drug *Abuse*, not Drug *Use*." While the political and scientific climates are quickly changing, there is still a significant way to go.

The United States is also largely responsible for the limited research throughout the rest of the world. Most of the available research studies on cannabis hail from Israel and the UK. There is a general belief perpetuated by the United States that cannabis is a drug of abuse, to be fought against rather than promoted and explored. The 1961 Single Convention on Narcotic Drugs requires all member states to keep cannabis illegal. While it still allows cannabis for medical and research purposes, its overall dismissal as a drug of abuse has limited this research ("U.N. Says").

If research had been encouraged and unrestricted rather than banned 70 years ago, so much more would be known about medicinal cannabis. The overwhelming anecdotal information that has accumulated in the shadows would instead have been revealed through rigorous clinical trials. Patients would not need to rely on the testimony of patient-researchers for data and practical guidance. However, this is reality as it is, and the world can no longer ignore the undeniable evidence of the therapeutic benefits that patients have reported over the past several years.

Patient Leaders

Most of the leaders in the cannabis extract movement were pulled in because they had to deal with their own illnesses. When someone is terribly sick, and no conventional pharmaceuticals will help them, he is forced to look for other options. For so many, cannabis has been the solution to their pain. After returning from the brink of death, several patients have been inspired to help others and the world as a whole.

The following list includes some of the most notable patients and physicians who have used their experiences to advance knowledge and assist others. While many of these individuals were not trained in formal scientific professions, their experiences and subsequent observations are powerful, credible, and completely supported by the existing scientific research. Their work should be used to influence further clinical trials.

RICK SIMPSON

The story of Rick Simpson is indispensable to the history of patient-led research and the realization of the higher-level healing capabilities of cannabis. Before Simpson, most people were only smoking cannabis or eating it in small quantities in the form of edibles. Through these methods, many people effectively relieved pain and symptoms of diseases, but virtually no one was reporting disease remission. Simpson showed that ingestion of concentrated cannabis oil is the best way to use cannabis medicinally and that doing so could directly treat various diseases. He is most notable for claiming that cannabis extracts could put virtually any cancer into remission. Thousands have used his protocol to treat their cancers.

Simpson was born in Springhill, Nova Scotia, on November 30, 1949 (Simpson). He was only 16 when he entered the workforce, and at 18 he began his career in power engineering. This was his lifelong endeavor until 1997, when a work-related head injury required him to leave his job. Shortly after, Simpson was diagnosed with post-concussion syndrome, which caused a number of symptoms such as tinnitus (ringing in the ears). Although he was prescribed numerous pharmaceuticals, none were effective.

In 1998, Simpson was introduced to the medicinal power of cannabis through a TV show called "The Nature of Things" with Dr. David Suzuki (Simpson). With no other options, Simpson acquired and tried smoking cannabis. He found it was more effective than any previous medications, so he sought out his doctor for a legal prescription. Simpson's physician refused to provide one, even after Simpson stated his intention to extract the oil from the cannabis. He initially wanted to use an extract as a means to avoid smoking, not knowing that doing so would also increase efficacy. Despite failing to acquire a prescription, Simpson continued to use cannabis and, through trial and error, developed a suitable method of extraction. In 2001, he ceased use of his prescription medications and began using only cannabis oil, which greatly improved his condition.

Simpson's own battle with cancer would lead him down the path to healing others. In late 2002, he was diagnosed with three skin cancers, two on his face and one on his chest (Simpson). One of these was removed surgically in January 2003. Before employing surgery for the other areas, Simpson decided to try cannabis oil. He knew of a 1974 study showing that THC could fight cancer, and he knew his oil had high levels of THC. Interestingly enough, the aforementioned study was concerned with lung cancer rather than skin cancer, but Simpson believed it was worth a shot. He placed his self-made cannabis oil on the cancers and covered them with bandages, and in four days they were gone.

Simpson's profound experience with cancer and his years-long previous experience treating post-concussion syndrome were enough to convince him of cannabis extract medicine's effectiveness. Without regard for the law, he began growing thousands of pounds of cannabis in his backyard and extracting it into oil (Simpson). Simpson gave away all the oil he produced at no cost to people in need. He soon found that the oil was working against nearly any condition he came across, including terminal forms of cancer, inflammatory and autoimmune disorders, diabetes, pain, nerve damage, and others. From several years of experience, he developed a protocol that consisted of ingesting 60 grams of cannabis oil in 90 days to treat most diseases.

On August 3, 2005, the Royal Canadian Mounted Police raided Simpson's home, confiscating 1,190 plants (Tetanish, "Seized"). Simpson claimed the actual number of plants confiscated was 1,620 (Simpson). He faced charges including possession of less than 30 grams of cannabis, possession of less than three kilograms of tetrahydrocannabinol for the purpose of trafficking, and unlawful production of cannabis.

At a sentencing hearing on November 30, 2007, Simpson faced penalties including a $2,000 fine, a firearms ban, and one-day custody deemed served by court appearance. Judge Felix Cacchione delivered the unusually light sentence because Simpson gave away the cannabis oil for free and held a sincere belief that he was helping people (Tetanish, "Simpson"). While awaiting the hearing, Simpson was arrested again for similar charges. Again, he received only a minor penalty, with Judge Carole Beaton providing almost the same reasoning as Judge Cacchione (King).

Rick Simpson's greatest contribution to the cannabis extract movement is the documentary *Run from the Cure*. The film, directed by Christian Laurette and released on February 10, 2008, detailed Simpson's work and the medicinal effects of cannabis oil (Laurette). It featured clips from

Simpson's appearances on news programs along with interviews from patients, including a terminal cancer survivor named James LeBlanc in full remission from using Simpson's oil. Other patients who experienced success with skin cancers or pain conditions were featured.

Despite Simpson's efforts in reaching out to government entities directly via letters and the public at large through his documentary, he initially was not taken seriously. Most people could not fathom the possibility that cannabis oil could treat not only so many cancers, but virtually any disease imaginable. For years, *Run from the Cure* was seen as a detriment and danger to the medicinal cannabis movement, as by exaggerating the potential of cannabis, the film might discredit its "real" benefits. Now the tables have turned, and not talking about the full capabilities of cannabis extracts is considered to be denying people lifesaving opportunities.

When Simpson began extracting and using cannabis oil, he did not know there were studies supporting every single observation he was seeing. He did not know that phytocannabinoids and our own endocannabinoids could kill almost any cancer cell imaginable. He did not know about the endocannabinoid system and the research that showed that manipulating it could indeed combat nearly any disease. Now that the science has become so much more prominent, and Simpson's observations have been replicated by doctors, dispensaries, corporations, and individuals across the world, his claims are taken more seriously.

While Simpson played a major role in launching the cannabis extract movement, he likely will not be the one to complete its goals. Other people have taken his work to the next level, greatly improving upon his dosing, production, and distribution methods. Many individuals with higher levels of formal education are better prepared to work with the next generation of cannabis extract medicines, producing consistent oils in laboratories and providing sophisticated dosage instructions based on the unique needs of patients. In the future, there will hopefully be a place for Rick Simpson, as he deserves to work in the industry he helped advance.

CORRIE YELLAND

Corrie Yelland is a terminal cancer survivor who used the information in *Run from the Cure* to save her own life. She has since become a leader in the cannabis extract movement, providing advice to people from across the world on how best to use cannabis oil. Before discussing her other work, it is important to become familiar with her healing experience.

Yelland's battle with health problems went beyond cancer. In May 2007, a heart attack led to heart surgery, which resulted in more than four years of chronic pain ("Corrie Yelland"). No amount of painkillers could reduce this pain, and sleeping pills were also ineffective for inducing any significant amount of sleep. In July 2011, she was diagnosed with anal canal cancer, and she also had two spots of skin cancer on her collarbone.

Surgery was attempted to remove the anal canal cancer. It was partially successful, but radiation was required to eliminate some remaining cancer ("Corrie Yelland"). Without this treatment, doctors gave Yelland two to six months to live. At this point, a friend sent Yelland the link to *Run from the Cure* ("Corrie Yelland"). After watching it, she was convinced that cannabis had real potential. This belief was bolstered further after she saw the sheer amount of research demonstrating how cannabinoids could fight cancer. In January 2012, Yelland began ingesting high–THC cannabis oil. She also applied the oil topically to her skin cancers, and they disappeared in just over a week.

In addition to using cannabis oil orally for the anal canal cancer, Yelland also utilized suppositories ("Corrie Yelland"). Getting cannabis oil as close as possible to the site of the cancer enhances potential results. By May 2012, an exam suggested that there was no more cancer, and a more thorough exam in September confirmed the cancer to be non-detectable.

Perhaps as importantly and remarkably, after only two weeks of ingesting cannabis oil, Yelland's constant and debilitating nerve pain disappeared ("Corrie Yelland"). She went from needing ten to fifteen Tylenol 3 (acetaminophen with codeine) daily, plus other painkilling drugs, to just half a Tylenol 3 within a 24-hour period. This change significantly improved Yelland's quality of life.

Since achieving remission from cancer, Corrie Yelland has become an extremely important source of help for new patients. Many people from around the world speak with her via Skype for advice related to cannabis oil. While she does not produce or provide cannabis oil directly, she often points people in the right direction for legally acquiring it.

As a result of speaking with so many people, she regularly reports the incredible successes she hears about through her Facebook page. She has posted dozens of successful accounts of patients whose cancer as well as a variety of difficult-to-treat diseases went into remission with the use of cannabis oil. In posts concerning cancer, Yelland will often close by saying something like, "Just in case you forgot … CANNABIS KILLS CANCER!" In posts related to other diseases, she will usually say, "Cannabis oil … for more than just cancers." She is also objective and shares information about cases in which cannabis oil failed to save lives, but in almost all cases there were still positive benefits. Yelland's fun and lively personality is a reminder of why each life is so important and must be saved.

Stan Rutner, John Malanca, and United Patients Group

Like Corrie Yelland, John Malanca, Corinne Malanca, and Stan Rutner turned a terrible situation into an opportunity to help thousands of other people around the world. Rutner was diagnosed with lung cancer that had metastasized to his brain in early 2011 (Hernandez). He began chemotherapy and radiation treatments in March 2011. These treatments were ineffective for Rutner's advanced cancer, and he entered hospice on August 12, 2011.

Rutner's son-in-law, John Malanca, suggested cannabis-infused coconut oil capsules as a way to help his father-in-law deal with pain (Hernandez). The positive effects turned out to extend way beyond analgesia. Rutner began using the capsules in November 2011, and in less than two weeks he was able to give up the 24/7 supplemental oxygen he had been required to use. He started sleeping better, gaining weight, and getting stronger. After about six months, Rutner added in high–THC and high–CBD cannabis oil, administered at different times, to increase anti-cancer activity. By January 27, 2013, scans revealed the tumors in his brain and lungs were no longer detectable (Hernandez).

After witnessing the remarkable, life-saving effects of cannabis oil, John and Corinne knew they had to do something to help others. They started United Patients Group, an organization dedicated to helping other patients acquire high-quality cannabis extracts. United Patients Group provides a wide variety of services to dispensaries and patients alike, including consulting and even emotional support.

Their role as an educational resource is also of paramount importance, and the website has an abundance of free information. When it comes to cannabis, there are so many different, varied issues to consider, such as the unique legal environments of different states, the respective availability of cannabis extracts, and the best ways to use cannabis medicines in different situations. For all these reasons, United Patients Group has become a truly valued resource for patients. They are respected by some of the top doctors, researchers, and activists in the cannabis extract movement.

Sharon Kelly

Sharon Kelly is one of the many patients United Patients Group has helped. She was diagnosed with Stage IV lung cancer on January 17, 2014, which had metastasized to at least three lymph nodes and the left collarbone (Kelly). Cancer was also detected in the left lung lining. At this point, there was nothing doctors could do to save her life, but chemotherapy had the potential to extend it. Her prognosis was grim and her life expectancy estimated between six and nine months.

Kelly had two intravenous chemotherapy sessions very shortly after diagnosis (Kelly). A test determined that she had a form of lung cancer that qualified her for Tarceva, an oral chemotherapeutic drug. She began this drug in February 2014. Doctors said, in the absolute best case, it might shrink the tumors slightly.

Kelly began looking for more effective alternatives and learned about the potential of cannabis medicine. She began ingesting high–THC cannabis oil orally as well as through a suppository method in order to maximize the amount of cannabinoids attacking the cancer (Kelly). In the beginning, she was also juicing cannabis leaves, which is an effective way to consume large quantities of raw, non-psychoactive cannabinoids. By September 3, 2014, the cancer had been completely eliminated.

Like other patients, Kelly is using her success to help others and give them hope. She attended the Inaugural Australian Medicinal Cannabis Symposium from November 21 to 22, 2014, where she informally shared her story with many attendees, including media. She has reached thousands of people through a YouTube video and makes herself completely available to anyone seeking help or information. This ripple effect from the healed helping others has significantly influenced the progress of cannabis extract medicine.

Samantha Wilkinson

Samantha Wilkinson is a multiple sclerosis patient living in Washington State who legally uses cannabis oil to manage her condition. She

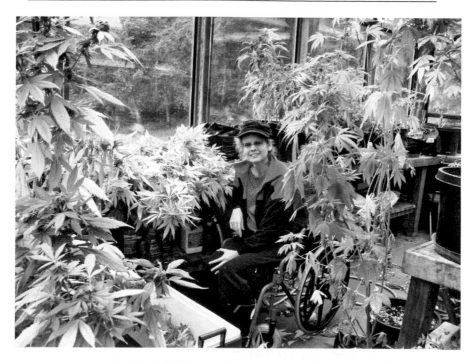

Sammy Jo Wilkinson (courtesy Doug Flomer).

was diagnosed at age 30 with a particularly devastating form of MS (Wilkinson). Conventional therapies damaged her heart, so she looked into medicinal cannabis as a treatment option. Wilkinson's husband, Doug, began growing and processing cannabis under Washington's medicinal cannabis law to ensure access to the highest-quality products.

Smoking cannabis was effective for Wilkinson, providing immediate relief from spasticity for two to three hours (Wilkinson). However, smoking was harsh on her lungs, and taking excessively large puffs could cause swooning. After learning about the enhanced potency of orally ingested cannabis extracts, which also avoided the need for smoking, Wilkinson decided to try them. Her husband first used isopropyl alcohol as the solvent, but switched to food-grade alcohol due to chemical aftertaste in the isopropyl-derived oil.

By using THC-rich and CBD-rich cannabis oils, Wilkinson can fine-tune her therapy for day or night. The myoclonic leg jerks that used to keep her awake half the night are a thing of the past (Wilkinson). The build-up of stiffness during the night, resulting in paralyzed legs by morning, is gone. She can bend her knees and move her legs in bed to prevent pressure-point pain. Extensor spasms are also gone; before, when she started to move, it could cause a violent full-body extension. With relief from stiffness and spasticity, her legs are easier to move and her daily exercise routine is up from 10 to 45 minutes. She has had more complete resolution from these symptoms with cannabis medicine than she ever achieved over the last 20 years with pharmaceutical drugs.

Samantha weighs 115 pounds and requires only two to three mg of THC per night. She mixes the THC-rich oil into a medium-chain triglyceride formula from coconut oil for easier dosing. Doing so also increases bioavailability. She takes higher doses of CBD cannabis oil and raw acidic cannabinoid preparations during the day, as there is no high. Wilkinson provides this example:

> Dosage Example:
> A 1ml syringe is equivalent to 1,000 mg of oil, but not 1,000 mg of THC
> If the cannabis oil is labeled 50 percent THC, multiplying 50 percent × 1,000mg oil = 500mg THC
> 1 oz of carrier oil is approximately 1,000 drops with an eye dropper
> 1 ml cannabis oil (500mg THC) dissolved in 1oz of carrier oil yields 0.5 mg THC per drop
> 2 drops = 1 mg THC
> 5 drops = 2.5 mg THC, so a 1 oz bottle = 200 doses
> (Wilkinson)

Wilkinson has shared her story so that others will benefit from her experience. Through careful preparation of high-quality extracts and close attention to dosing and responses, amazing healing can take place with cannabis.

Physician Leaders

There are many medical doctors at the forefront of cannabis medicine. While the full capabilities of extracts have largely been discovered by non-medical doctors, physicians have contributed substantially to the development of knowledge and the treatment of patients. It is highly unfortunate that, because of legal and cultural reasons, their greater participation has been impeded. Once cannabis is removed from Schedule I and extracts are treated like other drugs (or perhaps even less restricted), there will doubtless be an influx of doctors wanting to learn how to best use the "new" medicine.

It is important to point out that many doctors are not involved simply because their medical training did not cover the endocannabinoid receptor system or they went to medical school before the discovery of this system. After all, it is the endocannabinoid receptor system that is responsible for the amazing medicinal effects of cannabinoids, and understanding it is imperative to accepting cannabis as a genuine medicine. A survey by Dr. David Allen, a retired cardiothoracic and vascular surgeon, found that acceptance of cannabinoid science was startlingly low throughout the United States' 157 accredited medical schools (Allen). None of the schools taught this science as a course, and only 21 even mentioned it.

Despite the critical importance of the endocannabinoid system and its involvement in so many physiological functions, it is simply not taught to doctors. This is not surprising, given that the system was discovered in 1992 and there is a strong cultural bias against anything having to do with cannabis in the medical profession. Still, the lack of training is unfortunate and detrimental to the optimal practice of medicine.

DR. DONALD ABRAMS

One of the most accomplished doctors working with medicinal cannabis, if not the most successful, is Dr. Donald Abrams. He is the Chief of Hematology/Oncology at San Francisco General Hospital, as well as Professor of Clinical Medicine at the University of California San Francisco ("Donald Abrams"). He has held leadership roles in several other key positions.

Dr. Abrams is one of the only people who has conducted and continues to conduct federally approved cannabis research. As mentioned in the introduction, he had to fight extensively for permission to do formal research, but eventually he prevailed. One of his first studies was only approved because it proposed to examine a potential harm of cannabis in AIDS patients, but it turned out to be a clever way of indicating safety (Abrams et al., 258).

Dr. Abrams has received grants from the NIH for studying cannabis and HIV-related neuropathic pain, cannabis and opioids for treating cancer pain, and vaporization as a cannabis delivery system. His most recent and perhaps advanced trial will test vaporized CBD against pain resulting from sickle-cell anemia, a genetic disorder (Bloom). By working within the federal government's guidelines and carrying out gold-standard clinical trials, Dr. Abrams has been integral in proving the legitimacy of cannabis medicine.

While he has not carried out trials with cannabis and cancer, Dr. Abrams has expressed interest in doing so. In the Winter/Spring 2013 edition of *O'Shaughnessy's* journal, he discussed his thoughts on a clinical trial of cannabis oil combined with chemotherapy for glioblastoma patients (Gardner, "Doctors"). If the oil was shown to promote additional tumor reduction, it could be enough to justify a trial only using cannabis oil.

Dr. Abrams consulted on the case of Michelle Aldrich, a respected and longtime activist for medicinal cannabis (Gardner, "Doctors"). She was diagnosed with aggressive lung cancer and was able to eliminate it relatively quickly with a combination of chemotherapy and cannabis oil. Dr. Abrams commented, "The fact that Michelle didn't have cancer that could be located [after using the oil] is a bit unusual in someone who started treatment with an advanced stage disease. I don't usually see that in my patients. Did the cannabis oil make a difference? We don't know because we don't have a controlled study" (Gardner, "Doctors").

Once research on cannabis is expanded, Dr. Abrams may finally have the ability to study cannabis extracts for cancer in an appropriately controlled environment. Until then, he cautions people about foregoing traditional treatments for extracts. However, he is very supportive of cannabis use as an adjunct treatment, especially for side effects of chemotherapy and cancer-related pain ("The Science"). Dr. Abrams has found that even smoked cannabis is remarkably effective in five key areas: nausea elimination, appetite stimulation, pain reduction, sleep facilitation, and depression alleviation. Without cannabis, he would need to prescribe five drugs instead of a single natural plant.

One statement from Dr. Abrams sums up the indispensable nature of cannabis medicine. "As an oncologist, there is hardly a cancer patient that I see for whom I don't recommend cannabis" ("The Science"). It is tragic that, given such versatile utility, cannabis is not recommended or even allowed for more cancer patients.

DR. JEFFREY HERGENRATHER

As someone who has treated many severely ill patients with cannabis medicine, Dr. Jeffrey Hergenrather's experience is indispensable. He is the president of the Society of Cannabis Clinicians and vice president of the American Academy of Cannabinoid Medicine and has presented his findings at numerous CME-accredited conferences ("Dr. Jeffrey Hergenrather").

Before specializing in cannabis therapies, Dr. Hergenrather was a family practitioner. He now treats patients in all age ranges for a variety of diseases. At the Marijuana for Medical Professionals Conference, held September 9–11, 2014, he discussed his work with inflammatory bowel disease and late-stage Alzheimer's. The results in both cases were dramatic, with incredibly severe symptoms being significantly or almost completely alleviated with cannabis medicine.

Some of Dr. Hergenrather's presentations have described his work with cancer patients. He says that not all tumors are sensitive to cannabis, such as certain forms of lung and breast cancers (Futcher). However, skin cancers respond very well to topical treatment. Dr. Hergenrather has also seen effectiveness for neuroblastomas, hepatic, renal, pancreatic, colorectal, cervical, and prostate cancers, as well as several types of lymphomas and leukemias (Futcher). These remarkable observations demonstrate that while cannabis extracts are not perfect, they do work in many cases. With further research, it might be found that a different blend of phytochemicals in cannabis would be effective in some of the resistant cases.

Dr. David Bearman

One of the most prolific educators working with cannabis medicine is Dr. David Bearman. He has over forty years of experience in drug abuse treatment and has specialized in cannabis medicine for over ten years ("Home"). Dr. Bearman possesses an extensive understanding of the history behind cannabis and prohibition as a whole. By integrating his historical and medical knowledge, he can make a compelling case to nearly anyone about the utility of medicinal cannabis. Hundreds to thousands of individuals have directly benefited from his practice.

Dr. Bearman has presented his findings at hundreds of conferences, including those offering continuing medical education credits ("Speaker"). He has done more than most other practitioners to educate both lay audiences and other physicians about cannabis. Dr. Bearman appeared in the well-reviewed documentary *What If Cannabis Cured Cancer?* with other physicians, including Dr. Hergenrather. As the need for cannabis knowledge increases, he will likely become an even more important educator.

Dr. Dustin Sulak

Another very effective educator and practitioner is Dr. Dustin Sulak. He runs Integr8 Health in Maine, a health-care organization specializing in cannabis medicine and treating thousands of patients per year. Dr. Sulak is a Diplomat of the American Academy of Cannabinoid Medicine and has lectured nationally on medicinal cannabis, appearing at numerous CME-accredited medical conferences ("Medical Marijuana"). As a doctor of osteopathy, Dr. Sulak is particularly suited to using cannabis in ideal medical settings.

Several of Dr. Sulak's videos are available at no charge online; the content is remarkably extensive yet easy to comprehend. This makes his educational approach suitable for both laypersons and doctors alike. His extensive knowledge of the underlying science is the basis for his treatment of patients, and observations of "excellent clinical responses" continue to fuel his belief that cannabis is an excellent medicine.

Caregivers as Leaders

As discussed, the legal framework has created a situation in which caregivers have become leaders in cannabis medicine. Their treatment advice is founded on science and results from other patients. Until more formal clinical trials are conducted, this is all anyone can do. Thankfully, as the results show, even in this environment, the outcomes have been incredible.

There are many excellent caregivers involved in the cannabis movement; some of the best are discussed below. Unfortunately, given the overall nature of the cannabis industry, many unscrupulous individuals only concerned with profit are also involved. Further regulation of medicinal cannabis is necessary to ensure that caregivers are properly trained and meet the standards forward-thinking practitioners have created.

Mara Gordon

Arguably the most accomplished caregiver in the cannabis extract movement is Mara Gordon. She has presented at many of the CME-accredited conferences that several of the previously mentioned doctors have attended. Gordon specializes in the production of high-quality, lab-tested extracts and very consistent dosing protocols. All of her patients are required to undergo a rigorous intake process, as this is the only way to ensure that they are optimally treated. As a former consultant for Fortune 50 companies, her background in process engineering provided the skills necessary for this new line of groundbreaking work.

One of Gordon's most well-received presentations concerns five pediatric cancer cases. Her work has unequivocally demonstrated the amazing utility of carefully targeted cannabis extracts against the side effects of chemotherapy and cancers themselves. For example, parents of child brain cancer patients who were told that chemotherapy could at most stop the growth of tumors have seen nearly complete remissions by adding cannabis oil. These results are consistent with those from other caregivers, but Gordon's patients seem to respond especially well because of the close attention to dosing and nutritional strategies like cutting out sugar.

A unique strategy employed by Gordon involves treating patients with two strains—a high–THC extract and a high–CBD extract. By administering each extract at different times, the predominant cannabinoid can best do its job, while synergy between components is still achieved due to the whole-plant nature of the extracts.

Gordon is expected to be featured in a new documentary by Ricki Lake and Abby Epstein about the effectiveness of cannabis for killing cancer ("Weed People Movie"). The two primary patients featured are Sophie Ryan and Chico Ryder, both of whom had stunning success against optic pathway glioma and rhabdomyosarcoma respectively using Gordon's cannabis extract protocol. Sophie Ryan's case is even featured in *O'Shaugnessy's*, where her physician, Dr. Bonni Goldstein, remarks on the incredible progress and how chemotherapy was not expected to achieve those results (Goldstein).

In addition to children, Gordon has worked with hundreds of other patients for cancers and many diseases. In almost all cases, cannabis extracts have significantly benefited the health of her patients, even in cases where pharmaceuticals were largely ineffective.

CHRISTOPHER LARSON AND LAWRENCE RINGO

One of the most effective cannabis growers of all time was Lawrence Ringo. He was mostly if not entirely responsible for introducing high–CBD strains back into the medicinal cannabis community. In 2010, Ringo acquired the Sour Tsunami strain from Amsterdam. Through testing, the strain was identified as being a high–CBD variant. Ringo learned about the potential of CBD to alleviate diseases and began breeding projects to increase availability (Larson). He became known as a provider of high-quality medicines and even helped Tommy Chong beat prostate cancer with cannabis oil. Tragically, Ringo passed away on April 3, 2014, from lung cancer. His son Leroy carries on growing and improving the genetics (Larson).

Christopher Larson was Ringo's partner and another specialist in cannabis extraction and production. Together they founded the medicinal cannabis cooperative Lost Coast Botanicals in California, which dispenses only high–CBD cannabis products. Larson, who is highly regarded as a cannabidiol educator, has also continued Ringo's work and is a true expert in all topics related to cannabis medicine.

Larson's work has illuminated effective methods of safely utilizing cannabis extract medicine. He has found that a 1:1 THC:CBD oil, administered two to three times per day at 10–15 mg per dose, works well for autism, epilepsy, Parkinson's, and psychosis (Larson). Twenty to 25 percent of people cannot handle active THC due to anxiety, so CBD needs to be increased for them. The THC:CBD ratios and/or dosages should be titrated based on the patient's needs.

Results with cancer have also been positive. Larson has observed very good results with glioblastomas, including shrinking tumors with high–CBD, low–THC formulas. He has seen remission in three patients with Stage I or II cancers who used only cannabis oil and who have now been cancer-free for over two years (Larson). However, cannabis oil works very effectively when used in conjunction with traditional treatments and helps diminish their side effects.

DAVID MAPES

David Mapes is the proprietor behind Epsilon Research, which he founded in 2006. Mapes is a former professional chef and graduate of The Culinary Institute of America. Like many other producers, he became involved with cannabis after a serious injury, in 2004 (Mapes). His food-grade approach to manufacturing pure cannabis extracts derives from his training and experience.

Mapes conducts patient-level research using nutritional cannabis therapies, which have been effective in treating advanced cancers and chronic disorders. He has worked with more than 200 individuals and has observed a cancer success rate higher than that of conventional treatment (Mapes). The therapy advocated by Mapes includes using decarboxylated and raw acidic cannabinoids as well as high-quality nutrition.

In January 2014, Mapes released the *Epsilon Guide* series, a manual that anyone can use to produce extracts. It emphasizes the production of acidic cannabis extracts, which preserves raw compounds like THCA and CBDA. Mapes believes in the power of a raw-food diet for healing, and the use of cannabinoids is no exception. The first edition of the *Epsilon Guide* has been downloaded tens of thousands of times and is one of the foremost references for raw cannabinoid extraction (Mapes).

Summary

Thanks to the work of the individuals mentioned above and countless other activists, cannabis medicine has advanced considerably in the past several years. So much more is now known about the profound ways in which cannabis extracts can benefit patients beyond just palliative care. While clinical trials are still desperately needed, the data collected so far means we do not have to start from square one. If trials are informed by what we already know, they will be more effective and far more efficient.

Much like the cannabinoids themselves, leaders in the cannabis community have worked synergistically to increase knowledge and awareness. Similar observations between individuals of different backgrounds and educations lend credibility to what could easily be considered as grandiose claims, such as that cannabis extracts are able to directly treat all cancer. Patient-led research and observations are chiefly responsible for the dramatic rise in CBD availability and awareness. If not for these individuals accelerating change, it very well might have taken decades for mainstream scientific advocates to reach the same conclusions.

As the movement advances, there will no doubt be many other individuals who rise to leadership positions. The complex evolution of medicinal cannabis and its industry will not happen overnight, but it is up to everyone involved to remember why this medicine is so important and who is being helped. When sick patients are kept at the forefront of one's goals, the chances of success and making a meaningful impact are much higher.

Appendix: Resources

Educational Resources and Organizations

American Alliance for Medical Cannabis. Fellowship of health professionals, patients, educators, clergy, caregivers, and community members. Included in AAMC membership are experts in the field of cannabis medicine including clinical applications, cultivation, history, and medical preparations. www.letfreedomgrow.com

American Botanical Council. An independent, nonprofit research and education organization dedicated to providing accurate and reliable information for consumers, health care practitioners, researchers, educators, industry, and the media about the responsible use of herbs and medicinal plants. www.abc.herbalgram. org

American for Safe Access (ASA). An organization working to ensure safe and legal access to cannabis for therapeutic uses and research. www.safeaccessnow.org

California NORML. California's branch of the National Organization for the Reform of Marijuana Laws. www.canorml.org/cbd

The Canadian Consortium for the Investigation of Cannabinoids (CCIC). A nonprofit organization of basic and clinical researchers and health care professionals established to promote evidence-based research and education concerning the endocannabinoid system and therapeutic applications of endocannabinoid and cannabinoid agents. www.ccic.net

Cannabinoid Society. An organization founded by medical marijuana patients and doctors furthering the science of cannabinology through empirical data from scientific studies and clinical trials. www.cannabinoidsociety.com

Cannabis International Foundation. A resource for the dietary and medicinal use of cannabis. www.cannabisinternational.org

Citizens United for Research in Epilepsy (CURE). An organization dedicated to funding research for epilepsy. The website contains studies done on the effects of CBD on epilepsy. www.cureepilepsy.org

Coalition for Cannabis Policy Reform (CCPR). A nonpartisan organization dedicated to replacing the policy of cannabis prohibition with reasonable regulation, based on science, through ballot initiatives, legislative collaboration, and public education campaigns. www.cannabispolicyreform.org

Common Sense for Drug Policy (CSDP). A nonprofit organization dedicated to reforming drug policy and expanding harm reduction. www.csdp.org

Georgia Campaign for Access, Reform, and Education (C.A.R.E) Project. A volunteer

organization dedicated to the reform of Georgia's marijuana legislation. www.
gacareproject.com

International Association for Cannabis as Medicine. Association formed to advance
knowledge on cannabis, cannabinoids, the endocannabinoid system, and related
topics, especially with regard to their therapeutic potential. www.cannabis-med.
org

International Cannabinoid Research Society. The ICRS is a non-political, non-religious
organization dedicated to scientific research in all aspects of the cannabinoids,
ranging from biochemical, chemical, and physiological studies of the endogenous
cannabinoid system to studies of the abuse potential of recreational cannabis.
www.ircrs.co

Law Enforcement Against Prohibition (LEAP). A nonprofit organization of criminal
justice professionals who advocate for the legalization of marijuana. www.leap.cc

National Organization for the Reform of Marijuana Laws (NORML). NORML's mission
is to move public opinion sufficiently to legalize the responsible use of marijuana
by adults and to serve as an advocate for consumers to assure that they have access
to high-quality marijuana that is safe, convenient, and affordable. www.norml.
org

Project CBD. Nonprofit educational service dedicated to promoting and publicizing
research into the medical utility of cannabidiol (CBD) and other components of
the cannabis plant. www.projectcbd.org

Realm of Caring. Nonprofit organization formed to promote the use of concentrated
medicinal cannabis oil to treat debilitating illnesses, especially seizure disorders.
Affiliated with the distributors of Charlotte's Web cannabis strain. www.theroc.us

Unconventional Foundation for Autism (UF4A). Foundation dedicated to raising
awareness and advocating for nontraditional medicines and therapies to treat
autism. www.uf4a.com

The Wo/Men's Alliance for Medical Marijuana. A patient collective that provides information, facilitates education, and offers medical marijuana for patients with a
letter of recommendation from their physicians. www.wamm.org

Laboratory and Research Resources

California Pacific Medical Center Research Institute (CPMC). Medical research institute home to the McAllister lab, which focuses on the endocannabinoid system
and how it controls cell growth and programmed cell death, particularly in aggressive cancers. www.cpmc.org

CannLabs. A national provider of scientific methods and intellectual property for
assaying cannabis extracts. www.cannlabs.com

Center for Medicinal Cannabis Research (CMCR) at the University of California. The
purpose of the Center is to coordinate rigorous scientific studies to assess the
safety and efficacy of cannabis and cannabis compounds for treating medical conditions. Clinical trial results and links to videos on second opinions and treatment
options. www.cmcr.ucsd.edu/

Epsilon Research. Botanical research facility that offers case studies and clinical trials
to those who qualify for alternative medicines. www.epsilonresearch.com

Epsilon's Cannabis Extraction Guide available at http://www.epsilonresearch.org/#!
free-guide

International Cannabidiol Organization of Manufacturers and Research (ICOMR). Testing laboratories for CBD products for efficacy and toxic substances. www. icomr.org

Meda Biotech, LLC. A clinical-stage biopharmaceutical company developing a new class of hybrid water soluble drugs to help treat cancer, arthritis, and cardiovascular ailments. www.nanomeda.com

Pure Analytics. Cannabis lab services include analysis for cannabinoid content and potency level. www.pureanalytics.net

Science Daily Marijuana News. Daily updates on trial results and news concerning the use of cannabis in specific disorders. www.sciencedaily.com/news/mind_brain/marijuana/

Society of Cannabis Clinicians. Association of doctors who collect and evaluate research data in connection with clinical research programs pertaining to the use of medical marijuana. www.cannabisclinicians.org

Magazines

Big Buds. Online medical marijuana magazine containing news articles on the latest medical marijuana research and information. www.bigbudsmag.com

Canna Magazine. Magazine containing legislation news, global news, and scientific research articles on medical marijuana. www.cannamagazine.com

Cannabis Culture. Online news delivery about cannabis-related politics, activism, and growing information. www.cannabisculture.com

Cannabis Now. Bi-monthly print magazine containing economical, political, and legal information and articles on the legalization of marijuana.

CULTURE. Online magazine containing news and lifestyle trends of America's medical cannabis culture. www.ireadculture.com

420 Magazine. Magazine created to support the repeal of all cannabis prohibition laws and penalties. Includes news articles, product reviews, and fact-based research information on cannabis and its medical properties.

High Times. Marijuana-focused magazine that includes news, entertainment, videos, galleries, and growing information. www.hightimes.com

Recommended Books

Backes, Michael. 2014. *Cannabis Pharmacy: The Practical Guide to Medical Marijuana*. Evidence-based information on using cannabis for ailments and conditions.

Bello, Joan. 2011. *How Marijuana Cures Cancer*. A look into cancer, the cannibinoid system, and the effects of marijuana and/or its synthetic isomers on cancer.

British Medical Association. 1997. *Therapeutic Uses of Cannabis*. This book discusses the use and adverse effects of the drug for nausea, multiple sclerosis, pain, epilepsy, glaucoma, and asthma.

Conrad, Chris. 1997. *Hemp for Health: The Medicinal and Nutritional Uses of Cannabis Sativa*. This book discusses how marijuana relieves symptoms of glaucoma, epilepsy, migraines, insomnia, asthma, the nausea associated with AIDS and chemotherapy, and a host of other conditions.

Earleywine, Mitch. 2002. *Understanding Marijuana: A New Look at the Scientific Evidence.* This book examines the biological, psychological, and societal impact of marijuana.

Holland, Judy, editor. 2010. *The Pot Book: A Complete Guide to Cannabis—Its Role in Medicine, Politics, Science, and Culture.* A book containing contributions from experts in a number of medical disciplines, history, and the social sciences.

Joy, Janet, Stanley Watson, Jr., and John Benson, Jr., editors. 1999. *Marijuana and Medicine: Assessing the Science Base.* This book addresses the science base and therapeutic effects of marijuana for medical conditions such as glaucoma and multiple sclerosis.

Leonard-Johnson, Steven. 2014. *CBD-Rich Hemp Oil: Cannabis Medicine Is Back.* This book explores the similarities, differences, uses and benefits of hemp, cannabis, and medical marijuana, along with the interplay of THC and CBD.

Mack, Alison, and Janet Joy. 2000. *Marijuana as Medicine?* This book discusses the active compounds in marijuana and the prospects for developing medications using marijuana's active ingredients.

McVay, Doug, editor. 2014. *Drug War Facts.* An online book containing charts, facts and figures from government sources, government-sponsored sources, and peer-reviewed journals on public health and criminal justice issues pertaining to drug policies.

Ratsch, Christian. 2001. *Marijuana Medicine.* A comprehensive survey of the therapeutic, historical, and cultural uses of cannabis in traditions around the world.

Werner, Clint. 2011. *Marijuana Gateway to Health: How Cannabis Protects Us from Cancer and Alzheimer's Disease.* This book explains the benefits of using medical marijuana to treat brain tumors and Alzheimer's disease using information found from scientific research and studies.

Recommended Medical Journals

The American Journal of Medicine. A medical journal that publishes original clinical research of interest to physicians in internal medicine, both in academia and community-based practice. www.amjmed.com

Brazilian Journal of Medical and Biological Research. A medical journal that publishes the results of original research, which contributes significantly to knowledge in medical and biological sciences. www.scielo.br

Journal of the American Medical Association (JAMA). www.jama.jamanetwork.com/journal

Medical Cannabis Journal. Excellent resource for patients and practitioners on the historical and current uses of medical cannabis http://www.medicalcannabisjournal.net/

New England Journal of Medicine. A medical journal dedicated to bringing physicians research and key information at the intersection of biomedical science and clinical practice. www.nejm.org

Pharmacology and Therapeutics Journal. Medical journal that presents lucid, critical, and authoritative reviews of currently important topics in pharmacology. www.journals.elsevier.com/pharmacology-and-therapeutics/

The Weed Street Journal. Information on the medical use of cannabis, research, variations in strains, legal updates. www.theweedstreetjournal.com/

Websites and Additional Resources

Cannabis Extract Report. A comprehensive document integrating the scientific and anecdotal evidence demonstrating how cannabis extracts can fight cancer and control other diseases in humans. Includes medical documentation of terminal cancer patients in remission along with extensive analysis of scientific studies showing the anti-cancer potential of phytocannabinoids and endocannabinoids. www.cannabisextractreport.com

CBD Free For All. A project started with the goal of distributing free high–CBD cannabis clones/cuttings to any adult in Colorado who wishes to grow it for his own health. www.cbdfreeforall.org

Constance Pure Botanical Extract Resource. Information on cannabis; cannabis extracts recommended by oncologists. http://www.cbdfarm.org/

Cure Your Own Cancer. A website containing information on cannabis oil and its potential health benefits. This website includes scientific studies and user testimonials. www.cureyourowncancer.com

Elemental Wellness Center. Educational resource using laboratory analysis combined with ongoing research to better understand medical marijuana and its compounds. www.elementalwellnesscenter.com

Greenbridge Medical. A website detailing the work of Dr. Allen Frankel, who specializes in the use of medical marijuana. This website also includes research and information on the use of CBD to treat medical ailments. www.greenbridgemed.com

Grow Weed Easy. Online cannabis cultivation resource that suggests medical marijuana strains based on symptoms. www.growweedeasy.com

Leafly. An online directory for locating medical marijuana dispensaries. This website also contains scientific information on different strains of marijuana and their effects. www.leafly.com

The Mayo Clinic. A nonprofit worldwide leader in medical care, research, and education. www.mayoclinic.org

Medical Jane. A multifaceted resource that empowers medical marijuana patients and cannabis activists with industry news and information about strains, companies, events, and influential people in the industry. www.medicaljane.com

Medical Marijuana. An interactive online platform providing information on medical marijuana treatments, state and federal laws, and a list of medical marijuana dispensaries and doctors. www.medicalmarijuana.com

Medical Marijuana 411. This website features articles, bloggers, contributors and patient stories as well as scientific research on the use of medical marijuana. www.medicalmarijuana411.com

O'Shaughnessey's Reader. An ongoing history of the medical marijuana movement. This website features the "CBDiary," which details the effects of cannabidiol use. www.beyondthc.com

Stony Girl Gardens. A website detailing different strains of marijuana and their effects. This website also provides information on how to grow marijuana. www.gro4me.com

THC. An online library of medical case studies on the cannabis plant and the endocannabinoid system. www.thctotalhealthcare.com

United Patients Group. A website dedicated to providing discreet, professional, and safe resources for medical marijuana. www.unitedpatientsgroup.com

Blogs

Cannabis Law Group's Medical Marijuana Legal Blog. A blog ran by the Cannabis Law Group, which is a law firm dedicated to the rights of medical marijuana patients, collectives and growers. www.marijuanalawyerblog.com

Illegally Healed. This blog follows current events and news stories related to cannabis extract medicine. It features information on individual patients as well as large-scale developments. www.illegallyhealed.com

The Joint Blog. A blog designed to inform people on current cannabis news and information. www.thejointblog.com

Medical Marijuana Blog. A general information website containing information on state laws, doctors and dispensaries, recipes, and also a forum where users can discuss related topics. www.medicalmarijuanablog.com

Therapy in a Bottle. This website contains a blog written by the founder of the company "Therapy in a Bottle," which sells cannabis massage oil and other hemp-based products used for the purpose of pain relief for fibromyalgia and other chronic pain-inducing ailments. www.therapyinabottle.org

UK Cannabis Internet Activists. A cannabis law reform blog including a forum where people can openly discuss cannabis laws, personal stories, and other related information. www.ukcia.org

The Weed Blog. A blog dedicated to marijuana news and information, including grower tips, strain reviews, and legal news pertaining to marijuana. www.theweedblog.com

Government-Funded Medical Resources

National Cancer Institute. FAQ on the use of cannabis and cannabinoids in cancer. http://www.cancer.gov/cancertopics/pdq/cam/cannabis/patient/page2

National Cancer Institute. The Federal Government's principal agency for cancer research and training. The National Cancer Institute conducts and supports research, training, health information dissemination, and other programs with respect to the cause, diagnosis, prevention, and treatment of cancer, rehabilitation from cancer, and the continuing care of cancer patients and the families of cancer patients. www.cancer.gov

PubMed. The National Library of Medicine (NLM) at the National Institutes of Health (NIH). NLM search engine. The collective research components of the NIH with links to journal article abstracts and full-text articles. PubMed represents the largest biomedical research facility in the world. www.ncbi.nlm.nih.gov

Use of Cannabis Extracts in Seizure Disorders

American Epilepsy Society. Three studies presented at the American Epilepsy Society's 68th Annual Meeting offer new insights into diverse patient experiences with CBD. From Science Daily Marijuana News, Dec. 2014. www.sciencedaily.com/releases/2014/12/141208144146.htm

Compassionate Care NY. Medical Marijuana for People with Severe Epilepsy. Information on the use of cannabis extracts for seizure disorders. www.compassionatecareny.org/wp-content/uploads/MMJ-Epilepsy_March-24-14.pdf?7cb0fc

CURE Epilepsy: CBD in Seizure Disorders. Research news on the use of CBD in seizure disorders. www.cureepilepsy.org/research/cbd-and-epilepsy.asp

Epilepsy Foundation of Colorado. Treatment Options: The Use of Medical Marijuana or The Treatment of Epilepsy. www.epilepsycolorado.org/index.php?s=10784& item=5985

Jason and Jayden's Journey. Account of one of the first pediatric seizure disorder patients effectively treated with cannabis extracts. https://www.facebook.com/jasonand jaydensjourney

MedicalJane.com "Cannabis Classroom: The Role of Cannabis in Epilepsy and Seizure Disorders." July 3, 2014. http://www.medicaljane.com/2014/07/03/cannabis-class room-the-role-of-cannabis-in-epilepsy-and-seizure-disorders/

Medscape. "Seizure Disorders Enter Medical Marijuana Debate." Aug. 14, 2013. www. medscape.com/viewarticle/809434

Time Health News. "Finally, Some Hard Science on Medical Marijuana for Epilepsy Patients." Sept. 3, 2014. http://time.com/3264691/medical-marijauna-epilepsy-research-charlottes-web-study/

Use of Cannabis Extracts in Cancer

DrSircus.com. "Cannabis Cures Cancer," Sept. 2014. Information on government-funded research trials showing the benefits of THC and CBD oils in various types of cancer. http://drsircus.com/medicine/cannabis-cures-cancer

Medicalxpress.com. "Cannabis extract can have dramatic effect on brain cancer, says new research from St. George's, University of London." Nov. 17, 2014. http:// medicalxpress.com/news/2014-11-cannabis-effect-brain-cancer.html

Science Daily. Cannabis extract can have dramatic effect on brain cancer, says new research. Science Daily report from Nov. 2014 on the use of cannabis with radio-therapy. www.sciencedaily.com/releases/2014/11/141114085629.htm

Works Cited

Abel, Ernest L. *Marihuana: The First Twelve Thousand Years*. New York: Plenum Press, 1980.

Abrams, D.I., et al. "Cannabinoid–Opioid Interaction in Chronic Pain." *Clinical Pharmacology & Therapeutics* Dec. 2011: 844–851.

_____. "Short-Term Effects of Cannabinoids in Patients with HIV-1 Infection: A Randomized, Placebo-Controlled Clinical Trial." *Annals of Internal Medicine* 139.4 (2003): 258–266.

Aggarwal, Sunil K. "Cannabinergic Pain Medicine: A Concise Clinical Primer and Survey of Randomized-Controlled Trial Results." *The Clinical Journal of Pain* 29.2 (2013): 162–171.

Alberts, Bruce, et al. *Molecular Biology of the Cell*. New York: Garland Science, 2002.

Aldrich, Michael. "History of Therapeutic Cannabis." In *Cannabis in Medical Practice: A Legal, Historical and Pharmacological Overview of the Therapeutic Use of Marijuana*, edited by Mary Lynn Mathre, 35–55. Jefferson, NC: McFarland, 1997.

Alger, Bradley E. "Endocannabinoids and Their Implications for Epilepsy." *Epilepsy Currents* vol. 4(5) (2004): 169–173.

Allen, David. "Survey Shows Low Acceptance of the Science of the ECS." *Outword Magazine*, n.d., web, 3 Dec. 2014.

Amar, Mohamed. "Cannabinoids in Medicine: A Review of Their Therapeutic Potential." *Journal of Ethnopharmacology* 105. 1–2 (2006): 1–25.

Anson, Pat. "Marijuana Rated Most Effective for Treating Fibromyalgia." AmericanNewsReport. com, *National Pain Report*, Apr. 21, 2014.

Appendino, G., et al. "Antibacterial Cannabinoids from Cannabis Sativa: A Structure-Activity Study." *Journal of Natural Products* 71.8 (2008): 1427–1430.

Armentano, Paul. "Uh Oh: Politicians Formerly Against Medical Marijuana Now Singing Praises of Cannabidiol." www.alternet.org Feb. 21, 2014.

"Asset Forfeiture." DrugWarFacts.org., n.d. http://www.drugwarfacts.org/cms/forfeiture#sthash. GiauheGZ.dpbs.

Bachhuber, Marcus A., et al. "Medicinal Cannabis Laws and Opioid Analgesic Overdose Mortality in the United States, 1999–2010." *JAMA Internal Medicine* 174.10 (2014): 1668–1673.

Baker, David, et al. "The Therapeutic Potential of Cannabis." *The Lancet Neurology* 2.5 (May 2003): 291–298.

Beard, John. "The Action of Trypsin Upon the Living Cells of Jensen's Mouse-Tumor." *British Medical Journal* 1.2351 (1906): 140–141.

Bergamaschi, M.M., et al. "Cannabidiol Reduces the Anxiety Induced by Simulated Public Speaking in Treatment-Naïve Social Phobia Patients." *Neuropsychopharmacology* 36.6 (2011): 1219–1226.

_____. "Safety and Side Effects of Cannabidiol, a Cannabis Sativa Constituent." *Current Drug Safety* 6.4 (2011): 237–249.

Berman, J.S., et al. "Efficacy of Two Cannabis Based Medicinal Extracts for Relief of Central Neuropathic Pain from Brachial Plexus Avulsion: Results of a Randomised Controlled Trial." *Pain* 112.3 (2004): 299–306.

Besag, Frank. "Cognitive and Behavioral Outcomes of Epileptic Syndromes: Implications for Education and Clinical Practice." *Epilepsia* 47.s2 (2006): 119–125.

Bilkei-Gorzo, Andras. "The Endocannabinoid System in Normal and Pathological Brain Ageing." *Philosophical Transactions of the Royal Society B Biological Sciences* 367.1607 (2012): 3326–3341.

Bisogno, T., et al. "Molecular Targets for Cannabidiol and Its Synthetic Analogues: Effect on Vanilloid VR1 Receptors and on the Cellular Uptake and Enzymatic Hydrolysis of Anandamide." *British Journal of Pharmacology* 134(4) (2001): 845–852.

Bloom, Jonathan. "Study of Vaporized Medical Marijuana Treatment for Sickle Cell Anemia Given Green Light." ABC7News.com., Aug. 14, 2014.

Bluebird Botanicals. "About CBD Complete Oil." n.d., web, Aug. 14, 2014.

Borrelli, F., et al. "Beneficial Effect of the Non-Psychotropic Plant Cannabinoid Cannabigerol on Experimental Inflammatory Bowel Disease." *Biochemical Pharmacology* 85.9 (2013): 1306–1316.

_____. "Cannabidiol, a Safe and Non-Psychotropic Ingredient of the Marijuana Plant Cannabis Sativa, Is Protective in a Murine Model of Colitis." *Journal of Molecular Medicine* 87.11 (2009): 1111–1121.

Brady, C.M., et al. "An Open-Label Pilot Study of Cannabis-Based Extracts for Bladder Dysfunction in Advanced Multiple Sclerosis." *Multiple Sclerosis* 10.4 (2004): 425–433.

Buckley, Christine. "Hemp Produces Viable Biodiesel, UConn Study Finds." *UConn Today*. University of Connecticut, 6 Oct. 2010. http://today.uconn.edu/blog/2010/10/hemp-produces-viable-biodiesel-uconn-study-finds.

Bunam, Juliana. "Marijuana-Derived Epilepsy Drug in Clinical Trial for Children with Uncontrolled Seizures: UC San Francisco–Led Study First to Gather Data on Safety and Tolerability of Non-Psychotropic Component of Cannabis for Children." Press release from the University of California San Francisco, Feb. 3, 2014. http://www.ucsf.edu/news/2014/02/111641/marijuana-derived-epilepsy-drug-clinical-trial-children-uncontrolled-seizures.

Campos, A.C., "Cannabidiol Blocks Long-Lasting Behavioral Consequences of Predator Threat Stress: Possible Involvement of 5HT1A Receptors." *Journal of Psychiatric Research* 46.11 (2012): 1501–1510.

Campos, A.C., et al. "The Anxiolytic Effect of Cannabidiol on Chronically Stressed Mice Depends on Hippocampal Neurogenesis: Involvement of the Endocannabinoid System." *International Journal of Neuropsychopharmacology* 16.6 (2013): 1407–19.

_____. "Multiple Mechanisms Involved in the Large-Spectrum Therapeutic Potential of Cannabidiol in Psychiatric Disorders." *Philosophical Transactions of the Royal Society of London Biological Sciences* 367.1607 (2012).

"Cannabis for Infant's Brain Tumor, Doctor Calls Child 'A Miracle Baby.'" HuffingtonPost.com, Dec. 1, 2012.

Cano, Carla E., et al. "Nupr1: The SwissKnife of Cancer." *Journal of Cellular Physiology* 226.6 (2011): 1439–1443.

Carter, Gregory T., et al. "Cannabis in Palliative Medicine: Improving Care and Reducing Opioid-Related Morbidity." *American Journal of Hospice and Palliative Medicine* 28.5 (2011): 297–303.

Cha, Ariana. "Marijuana Research Hampered by Access from Government and Politics, Scientists Say." *The Washington Post*, Mar. 21, 2014.

Chagas, M.H., et al. "Cannabidiol Can Improve Complex Sleep-Related Behaviours Associated with Rapid Eye Movement Sleep Behaviour Disorder in Parkinson's Disease Patients: A Case Series." *Journal of Clinical Pharmacy and Therapeutics* 39.5 (2014): 564–566.

Chagas, M.H., et al. "Effects of Cannabidiol in the Treatment of Patients with Parkinson's Disease: An Exploratory Double-Blind Trial." *Journal of Psychopharmacology* (Oxford) 28.11 (2014): 1088–1098.

Chen, T., et al. "The Isolation and Identification of Two Compounds with Predominant Radical

Scavenging Activity in Hempseed (Seed of Cannabis Sativa L.)." *Food Chemistry* 134.2 (2012): 1030–1037.

Cheng, D., et al. "Chronic Cannabidiol Treatment Improves Social and Object Recognition in Double Transgenic APPswe/PS1ΔE9 Mice." *Psychopharmacology* (Berl) 231.15 (2014): 3009–3017.

Cilio, Maria Roberta, et al. "The Case for Assessing Cannabidiol in Epilepsy." *Epilepsia*, May 22, 2014: n.p.

Clarke, Robert C. *Marijuana Botany, An Advanced Study: The Propagation and Breeding of Distinctive Cannabis.* Oakland, CA: Ronan Publishing, 1981.

_____, and David Paul Watson. "Botany of Natural Cannabis Medicines." In *Cannabis and Cannabinoids: Pharmacology, Toxicology, and Therapeutic Potential*, edited by Franjo Grotenhermen and Ethan Russo, 3–13. Binghamton, NY: Haworth Integrative Healing Press, 2002.

_____, and Mark D. Merlin. *Cannabis Evolution and Ethnobotany.* Berkeley: University of California Press, 2013.

Conrad, Chris. *Hemp for Health: The Medicinal and Nutritional Uses of Cannabis Sativa.* Rochester: Healing Arts Press, 1997.

Corderoy, Amy. "Cannabis May Help Reverse Dementia: Study." *Sydney Morning Herald*, Feb. 6, 2013.

"Corrie Yelland | CannabisNationRadio.com | Cannabis Marijuana & Hemp News." Cannabis NationRadio.com, Jan. 11, 2013.

Courtney, William. "Origins of Cannabis International Foundation." Cannabis International Website, 2004.

Crippa, J.A., et al. "Neural Basis of Anxiolytic Effects of Cannabidiol (CBD) in Generalized Social Anxiety Disorder: A Preliminary Report." *Journal of Psychopharmacology* (Oxford) 25.1 (2011): 121–130.

Croxford, J.L. "Therapeutic Potential of Cannabinoids in CNS Disease." *CNS Drugs* 17.3 (2003): 179–202.

Cunha, Jomar M., et al. "Chronic Administration of Cannabidiol to Healthy Volunteers and Epileptic Patients." *Pharmacology* 21(3) (1980): 175–185. http://www.ncbi.nlm.nih.gov/pub med/7413719.

"DEA Clarifies Status of Hemp in the Federal Register." *United States Drug Enforcement Administration Press Release*, Oct. 9, 2001.

De Filippis, D., et al. "Cannabidiol Reduces Intestinal Inflammation Through the Control of Neuroimmune Axis." *PLoS ONE* 6.12 (2011): e28159.

DeGrandpre, Richard. *The Cult of Pharmacology: How America Became the World's Most Troubled Drug Culture.* Durham, NC: Duke University Press, 2006.

De Petrocellis, L., et al. "Non-THC Cannabinoids Inhibit Prostate Carcinoma Growth in Vitro and in Vivo: Pro-Apoptotic Effects and Underlying Mechanisms." *British Journal of Pharmacology* 168.1 (2013): 79–102.

Deshpande, Laxmikant S., et al. "Endocannabinoids Block Status Epilepticus in Cultured Hippocampal Neurons." *European Journal of Pharmacology*, Mar. 8, 2007: 52–59. http://www.ncbi.nlm.nih.gov/pmc/articles/PMC2617750/.

Devinsky, Orrin, et al. "Cannabidiol: Pharmacology and Potential Therapeutic Role in Epilepsy and Other Neuropsychiatric Disorders." *Epilepsia*, June 2014. http://onlinelibrary.wiley.com/doi/10.1111/epi.12631/full.

Dodd, Beth. "Medical Refugees Flock to Colorado." *The Mountain Jackpot* 10(12) (2014): 1, 10–11.

"Donald Abrams | UCSF Profiles." Ucsf.edu. University of California, San Francisco, n.d.

"Dr. Jeffrey Hergenrather." MedicalJane.com. Medical Jane, n.d.

Drug Enforcement Agency. "2012 Domestic Cannabis Eradication/Suppression Statistical Report." n.d., n.p.

Durst, R., et al. "Cannabidiol, a Nonpsychoactive Cannabis Constituent, Protects Against Myocardial Ischemic Reperfusion Injury." *Heart and Circulatory Physiology* 293.6 (2007): H3602–H3607.

Earleywine, Mitch. *Understanding Marijuana: A New Look at the Scientific Evidence.* New York: Oxford University Press, 2012.

El-Alfy, A.T., et al. "Antidepressant-Like Effect of Delta9-Tetrahydrocannabinol and Other Cannabinoids Isolated from Cannabis Sativa L." *Pharmacology Biochemistry and Behavior* 95.4 (2010): 434–442.

Elmore, Susan. "Apoptosis: A Review of Programmed Cell Death." *Toxicologic Pathology* 35.4 (2007): 495–516.

ElSohly, Mahmoud A. "Chemical Constituents of Cannabis." *Cannabis and Cannabinoids: Pharmacology, Toxicology, and Therapeutic Potential,* edited by Franjo Grotenhermen and Ethan Russo, 27–36. Binghamton, NY: Haworth Integrative Healing Press, 2002.

Esposito, G., et al. "Cannabidiol in Vivo Blunts Beta-Amyloid Induced Neuroinflammation by Suppressing IL-1beta and iNOS Expression." *British Journal of Pharmacology* 151.8 (2007): 1272–1279.

_____. "Cannabidiol Reduces Aβ-Induced Neuroinflammation and Promotes Hippocampal Neurogenesis Through PPARγ Involvement." *PLoS ONE* 6.12 (2011): e28668.

Fankhauser, Manfred. "History of Cannabis in Western Medicine." In *Cannabis and Cannabinoids: Pharmacology, Toxicology, and Therapeutic Potential*, edited by Franjo Grotenhermen and Ethan Russo, 37–51. Binghamton, NY: Haworth Integrative Healing Press, 2002.

Fernandez-Ruiz, J., M. Moreno-Martet, C. Rodriguez-Cueto, C. Palomo-Garo, and M. Gomez-Canas, et al. "Prospects for Cannabinoid Therapies in Basal Ganglia Disorders." *British Journal of Pharmacology* 163.7 (2011): 1365–1378.

Ferner, Matt. "Congress Passes Historic Medical Marijuana Protections in Spending Bill." *The Huffington Post*, Dec. 14, 2014.

Ferretti, C., et al. "Molecular Circuits Shared by Placental and Cancer Cells, and Their Implications in the Proliferative, Invasive and Migratory Capacities of Trophoblasts." *Human Reproduction Update* 13.2 (2007): 121–141.

Fine, Doug. "Hemp Is on Its Way to Your Car Battery and Many Things You Haven't Yet Imagined." AlterNet.org, Oct. 14, 2014. http://www.alternet.org/drugs/hemp-its-way-your-car-battery-and-many-things-you-havent-yet-imagined.

Fine, Perry G., et al. "The Endocannabinoid System, Cannabinoids, and Pain." *Rambam Maimonides Medical Journal* 4.4 (2013): e0022.

Fox, Steve, et al. *Marijuana Is Safer: So Why Are We Driving People to Drink?* White River Junction, VT: Chelsea Green Press, 2013.

Frankel, Allan. "Cannabis Oils." *Greenbridge Medical Center Website.* Greenbridge Medical Center, Mar. 9, 2013.

Fusar-Poli, P., et al. "Distinct Effects of Delta-9-Tetrahydrocannabinol and Cannabidiol on Neural Activation During Emotional Processing." *Archives of General Psychiatry* 66.1 (2009): 95–105.

Futcher, Jane. "Cannabis Physician Presents Treatment Successes at Laytonville Garden Club." Willitsnews.com. *Willits News*, 4 Jul. 2014.

Gallily, Ruth, et al. "γ-Irradiation Enhances Apoptosis Induced by Cannabidiol, a Non-Psychotropic Cannabinoid, in Cultured HL-60 Myeloblastic Leukemia Cells." *Leukemia & Lymphoma* 44.10 (2003): 1767–1773.

Galvan, Astrid. "Fired Professor Suzanne Sisley Isn't Giving Up on Marijuana Research." *The Huffington Post*, July 20, 2014.

Gamonski, William. "Harness the Nutritional Power of Hemp Seeds." *Life Extension*, (July 2014): 93–6.

García, C., et al. "Symptom-Relieving and Neuroprotective Effects of the Phytocannabinoid Δ⁹-THCV in Animal Models of Parkinson's Disease." *British Journal of Pharmacology* 163.7 (2011): 1495–1506.

García-Arencibia, M., et al. "Evaluation of the Neuroprotective Effect of Cannabinoids in a Rat Model of Parkinson's Disease: Importance of Antioxidant and Cannabinoid Receptor-Independent Properties." *Brain Research* 1134.1 (2007): 162–170.

Gardner, Fred. "Doctors Stress Need to Document Anti-Cancer Effects of Cannabis 'Oil.'" BeyondTHC.com. *O'Shaughnessy's*, Winter/Spring 2013.

_____. "Realm of Caring Comes to California." *O'Shaugnessy's*, print edition, Feb. 28, 2014.

Gedde, Margaret, and Edward Maa. "Whole Cannabis Extract of High Concentration Cannabidiol May Calm Seizures in Highly Refractory Pediatric Epilepsies." *In Press with the American Epilepsy Society*, 67th Annual Meeting, December 6–10, 2013: 1.

Gehringer, Dale. "Inside the DEA." *Reason Magazine*, December 1986.

Goffin, Karolien, et al. "In Vivo Activation of Endocannabinoid System in Temporal Lobe Epilepsy with Hippocampal Sclerosis." *Brain* 134(4) (2011): 1033–1040.

Goldstein, Bonni. "Cannabis vs. Glioma: Another Encouraging 'Anecdote.'" BeyondTHC.com. *O'Shaugnessy's*, Jun. 20, 2014.

_____. "Dr. Goldstein on Caring for Kids with Epilepsy." *O'Shaugnessy's* Print Edition, Feb. 24, 2014.

Goodman, Louis, and Alfred Gilman, eds. *Goodman & Gilman's The Pharmacological Basis of Therapeutics*, Second Edition. New York: MacMillan, 1955.

_____, and _____. *Goodman & Gilman's The Pharmacological Basis of Therapeutics*, Eleventh Edition. New York: MacMillan, 2006.

Goodman, Neil. "An Overview of the Endogenous Cannabinoid System, Its Components and Possible Roles of This Recently Discovered Regulatory System." *Erowid Cannabis Vaults Pharmacology*, April 2011. https://www.erowid.org/plants/cannabis/cannabis_pharmacology 2.shtml.

Gray, Mike. "The Devil Weed and Harry Anslinger." *Common Sense for Drug Policy*. Public Service Announcement, 2006.

Green, Greg. *The Cannabis Grow Bible*, 2nd Edition. San Francisco: Green Candy Press, 2010.

Grimaldi, C., et al. "Anandamide Inhibits Adhesion and Migration of Breast Cancer Cells." *Experimental Cell Research* 312.4 (2006): 363–373.

Grinspoon, Lester. "Cannabinopathic Medicine: An Update to Whither Medical Marijuana." *Contemporary Drug Problems*, vol. 27 (Spring 2000).

_____. "Medical Marijuana: A Note of Caution Primum non nocere." *O'Shaugnessy's: The Journal of Cannabis in Clinical Practice*, Summer 2009.

_____, and James Bakalar. *Marihuana the Forbidden Medicine*, Revised and Expanded Edition. New Haven, CT: Yale University Press, 1997.

Grlic, L. "A Comparative Study on Some Chemical and Biological Characteristics of Various Samples of Cannabis Resin." *Bulletin on Narcotics*, vol. 14 (1976): 37–46.

Grotenhermen, Franjo, and Ethan Russo, eds. *Cannabis and Cannabinoids: Pharmacology, Toxicology, and Therapeutic Potential*. Binghamton, NY: Haworth Integrative Healing Press, 2002.

Gupta, Sanjay. "Why I Changed My Mind on Weed." CNN.com. Cable News Network, Aug. 8, 2013. http://www.cnn.com/2013/08/08/health/gupta-changed-mind-marijuana.

Guzmán, M., et al. "A Pilot Clinical Study of Δ9-tetrahydrocannabinol in Patients with Recurrent Glioblastoma Multiforme." *British Journal of Cancer* 95.2 (2006): 197–203.

"GWPharma—GW Pharmaceuticals Announces Physician Reports of Epidiolex® Treatment Effect in Children and Young Adults with Treatment-Resistant Epilepsy from Physician-Led Expanded Access Treatment Program." GWPharm.com. GW Pharmaceuticals, 17 Jun. 2014.

"GW Pharmaceuticals plc Announces US Patent Allowance for Use of Cannabinoids in Treating Glioma." GWPharm.com. GW Pharmaceuticals, 11 Dec. 2013.

Haglage, Abby. "Judge Could Smash Marijuana Law." *The Daily Beast*, Nov. 4, 2014.

Hanahan, Douglas, and Robert A. Weinberg. "Hallmarks of Cancer: The Next Generation." *Cell* 144.5 (2011): 646–674.

Herer, Jack. *The Emperor Wears No Clothes*, 12th Edition. Austin, TX: Ah Ha Press, 2010.

"Hergenrather Presents Study of Crohn's Patients as a Template for Clinical Research on Cannabis." BeyondTHC.com. *O'Shaugnessy's*, Aug. 2013.

Herkenham, M., et al. "Cannabinoid Receptor Localization in Brain." *Proceedings of the National Academy of Science* 87.5 (1990): 1932–1936.

Herman, T.S., et al. "Nabilone: A Potent Antiemetic Cannabinol with Minimal Euphoria." *Biomedicine* 27.9–10 (1977): 331–334.

Hernandez, Roberto C. "Convinced of the Cure." IReadCulture.com. *CultureMag*, 6 Sep. 2013.

Hill, A.J., et al. "Cannabidivarin Is Anticonvulsant in Mouse and Rat." *British Journal of Pharmacology* (Dec. 2012): 1629–1642.

Hill, T.D., et al. "Cannabidivarin-Rich Cannabis Extracts are Anticonvulsant in Mouse and Rat via a CB1 Receptor-Independent Mechanism." *British Journal of Pharmacology* 170.3 (2013): 679–692.

Hofmann, Mackenzie E., and Charles J. Frazier. "Marijuana, Endocannabinoids, and Epilepsy: Potential and Challenges for Improved Therapeutic Intervention." *Experimental Neurology* vol. 244 (2013): 43–50.

"Home." DavidBearmanMD.com. DavidBearmanMD.com, n.d. 3 Dec. 2014.

Howelett, A.C., et al. "International Union of Pharmacology. XXVII. Classification of Cannabinoid Receptors." *Pharmacological Reviews*, (June 2002):161–201. http://intl.pharmrev.org/content/54/2/161.full.

Huestis, Marilyn. "Human Cannabinoid Pharmacokinetics." *Chemistry and Biodiversity* 4.8 (2007): 1770–1804.

Ibrahim, Mohab M., et al. "CB2 Cannabinoid Receptor Activation Produces Antinociception by Stimulating Peripheral Release of Endogenous Opioids." *Proceedings of the National Academy of Sciences of the United States of America* 102.8 (2005): 3093–3098.

Ingold, John. "Lawmakers in 11 States Approve Low-THC Medical Marijuana Bills." *The Denver Post*, June 30, 2014. http://www.denverpost.com/marijuana/ci_26059454/lawmakers-11-states-approve-low-thc-medical-marijuana.

"Insys Therapeutics Receives FDA Orphan Drug Designation for Its Pharmaceutical Cannabidiol as a Potential Treatment for Glioma." Marketwatch.com. *MarketWatch*, 29 Sep. 2014.

Iuvone, T., et al. "Neuroprotective Effect of Cannabidiol, a Non-Psychoactive Component from Cannabis Sativa, on Beta-Amyloid-Induced Toxicity in PC12 Cells." *Journal of Neurochemistry* 89.1 (2004): 134–141.

Jackman, Tom. "Northern Va. Families Move to Colorado to Get Medical Marijuana for Children with Epilepsy." WashingtonPost.com. *Washington Post*, 12 Apr. 2014.

Jiang, Hong-En, et al. "A New Insight into Cannabis Sativa (Cannabaceae) Utilization from 2500-year-old Yanghai Tombs, Xinjang, China." *Journal of Ethnopharmacology* 105.3 (2006): 414–422.

Johnson, J.R., et al. "Multicenter, Double-Blind, Randomized, Placebo-Controlled, Parallel-Group Study of the Efficacy, Safety, and Tolerability of THC:CBD Extract and THC Extract in Patients with Intractable Cancer-Related Pain." *Journal of Pain and Symptom Management* 39.2 (2010): 167–179.

Jones, Nicholas A., et al. "Cannabidiol Displays Antiepileptiform and Antiseizure Properties in Vitro and in Vivo." *Journal of Pharmacology and Experimental Therapeutics*, Feb. 2010: 569–577.

_____. "Cannabidiol Exerts Anti-convulsant Effects in Animal Models of Temporal Lobe and Partial Seizures." *Seizure*, June 2012: 344–352.

Joy, J., S. Watson, and J. Benson, eds. "Marijuana and Medicine: Assessing the Science Base." *Institute of Medicine*. Washington, DC: The National Academies Press, 1999.

Kalant, Harold. "Medicinal Use of Cannabis: History and Current Status." *Pain Research and Management* (2001): 80–94.

Kano, Masanobu. "Control of Synaptic Function by Endocannabinoid-Mediated Retrograde Signaling." *Proceedings of the Japan Academy*, Series B (2014): 235–250.

Kano M., et al. "Endocannabinoid-mediated Control of Synaptic Transmission." *Physiological Reviews* (2009): 309–380.

Kapalos, Helen. "Cannabis Oil: Raided for Helping Their Son." Au.news.yahoo.com., Aug. 3, 2014.

Karler, R., et al. "The Anticonvulsant Activity of Cannabidiol and Cannabinol." Life Sciences 13.11 (1973): 1527–1531.

Kelly, Sharon. Personal Interview, 21 Nov. 2014.

King, Bonnie. "Man Heralded for Curing Cancer Seeks Asylum in Europe." Salem-News.com., 5 Dec. 2009.

Kleiner, D., and K. Ditrói. "The Potential Use of Cannabidiol in the Therapy of Metabolic Syndrome." *Orvosi Hetilap* 153.13 (2012): 499–504.

Kozela, E., et al. "Cannabinoids Decrease the th17 Inflammatory Autoimmune Phenotype." *Journal of Neuroimmune Pharmacology* 8.5 (2013): 1256–1276.

Kuipers, Dean. *Burning Rainbow Farm: How a Stoner Utopia Went Up in Smoke*. New York: Bloomsbury Publishing, 2006.

Lafourcade, M., et al. "Nutritional Omega–3 Deficiency Abolishes Endocannabinoid-Mediated Neuronal Functions." *Nature Neuroscience* 14.3 (2011): 345–350.

Larson, Christopher. Personal Interview, 18 Dec. 2014.

"Latest Facts and Figures." Alz.org., Alzheimer's Association.

Laurette, Christian. *Run from the Cure*. February 10, 2008. https://archive.org/details/Run-FromTheCure-PhoenixTearsMovie.

Lee, Martin A. "The Cannabis Health Revolution: Understanding and Utilizing the Latest Science and Research." Session 3, online course, 6 Aug. 2014.

_____. "The 'CBD Only' Stampede." *Project CBD*, 22 Mar. 2014.

_____. "How CBD Works." *O'Shaughnessy's*, Autumn 2011.

_____. *Smoke Signals: A Social History of Marijuana—Medical, Recreational and Scientific*. New York: Scribner, 2012.

_____, and Valerie Corral. "The Cannabis Health Revolution: Understanding and Utilizing the Latest Science and Research." Session 5, online course, 20 Aug. 2014.

_____, and Jahan Marcu. "The Cannabis Health Revolution: Understanding and Utilizing the Latest Science and Research." Session 2, online course, 30 Jul. 2014.

_____, and Michelle Sexton. "The Cannabis Health Revolution: Understanding and Utilizing the Latest Science and Research." Session 1, online course, 23 Jul. 2014.

_____, and Dustin Sulak. "The Cannabis Health Revolution: Understanding and Utilizing the Latest Science and Research." Session 4, online course, 13 Aug. 2014.

Legault, J., and A. Pichette. "Potentiating Effect of Beta-Caryophyllene on Anticancer Activity of Alpha-Humulene, Isocaryophyllene and Paclitaxel." *Journal of Pharmacology and Pharmacotherapeutics* 59.12 (2007): 1643–1647.

Leigh, Vivien. "Maine Becoming Home to Marijuana Refugee Families." WCSH6.com. Gannett Satellite Information Network, May 21, 2014.

Leweke, F.M., et al. "Cannabidiol Enhances Anandamide Signaling and Alleviates Psychotic Symptoms of Schizophrenia." *Translational Psychiatry* (2012): e94.

Li, H.L. "An Archaeological and Historical Account of Cannabis in China." *Economic Botany* 28.4 (1974): 437–448.

_____. "The Origin and Use of Cannabis in Asia: Linguistic and Cultural Implications." *Economic Botany* 28.3 (1973): 293–301.

Ligresti, A., et al. "Antitumor Activity of Plant Cannabinoids with Emphasis on the Effect of Cannabidiol on Human Breast Carcinoma." *Journal of Pharmacology and Experimental Therapeutics* 318.3 (2006): 1375–1387.

Ludányi A., et al. "Downregulation of the CB1 Cannabinoid Receptor and Related Molecular Elements of the Endocannabinoid System in Epileptic Human Hippocampus." *The Journal of Neuroscience* (2008): 2976–2990.

Ludlow, Fitz Hugh. *The Hasheesh Eater: Being Passages from the Life of a Pythagorean*. New York: Harper, 1857.

Lutz, Beat. "On-demand Activation of the Endocannabinoid System in the Control of Neuronal Excitability and Epileptiform Seizures." *Biochemical Pharmacology* (2004): 1691–1698. http://www.ncbi.nlm.nih.gov/pubmed/15450934.

_____. "Physiological and Pathological Functions of the Endocannabinoid System in the Central Nervous System" *CMR Journal* (2008).

Lynch, Mary E., and Fiona Campbell. "Cannabinoids for Treatment of Chronic NonCancer Pain: A Systematic Review of Randomized Trials." *British Journal of Clinical Pharmacology* 72.5 (2011): 735–744.

Maa, Edward, and Paige Figi. "The Case for Medical Marijuana in Epilepsy." *Epilepsia* (2014): 783–786.

Maccarone, Mauro, et al. "Anandamide Induces Apoptosis in Human Cells via Vanilloid Receptors." *The Journal of Biological Chemistry* 275.41 (2000): 31938–31945.

_____. "Cannabinoid Receptor Signalling in Neurodegenerative Diseases: A Potential Role for Membrane Fluidity Disturbance." *British Journal of Pharmacology* 163.7 (2011): 1379–1390.

Mackie, Kenneth. "Understanding Cannabinoid Psychoactivity with Mouse Genetic Models." *PLoS Biology* 5.10 (2007): 2106–2108.

Maione, S., et al. "Non-Psychoactive Cannabinoids Modulate the Descending Pathway of Antinociception in Anaesthetized Rats Through Several Mechanisms of Action." *British Journal of Pharmacology* 162.3 (2011): 584–596.

Mapes, David. Personal Interview, 26 Dec. 2014.

Marcu, J.P., et al. "Cannabidiol Enhances the Inhibitory Effects of Delta9-Tetrahydrocannabinol on Human Glioblastoma Cell Proliferation and Survival." *Molecular Cancer Therapeutics* 9.1 (2010): 180–189.

"Marijuana Fact Sheet." Office of Drug Control Policy, The White House.

Martin, Billy R., and Aron H. Lichtman. "Cannabinoid Transmission and Pain Perception." *Neurobiology of Disease* 5.6 (1998): 447–461.

Massi, Paola, et al. "Antitumor Effects of Cannabidiol, a Nonpsychoactive Cannabinoid, on Human Glioma Cell Lines." *Journal of Pharmacology and Experimental Therapeutics* 308.3 (March 2004): 838–845.

_____. "Cannabidiol as Potential Anticancer Drug." *British Journal of Clinical Pharmacology* 75.2 (2013): 303–312.

_____. "The Non-Psychoactive Cannabidiol Triggers Caspase Activation and Oxidative Stress in Human Glioma Cells." *Cellular and Molecular Life Sciences* 63.17 (2006): 2057–2066.

Mathern, Gary, et al. "From the Editors: Cannabidiol and Medical Marijuana for the Treatment of Epilepsy." *Epilepsia* (2014).

Mathre, Mary Lynn, ed. *Cannabis in Medical Practice: A Legal, Historical and Pharmacological Overview of the Therapeutic Use of Marijuana.* Jefferson, NC: McFarland, 1997.

McAllister, Sean, et al. "Cannabidiol as a Novel Inhibitor of Id-1 Gene Expression in Aggressive Breast Cancer Cells." *Molecular Cancer Therapeutics* 6.11 (2007): 2921–2927.

_____. "Pathways Mediating the Effects of Cannabidiol on the Reduction of Breast Cancer Cell Proliferation, Invasion, and Metastasis." *Breast Cancer Research and Treatment* 129.1 (2011): 37–47.

McKallip, Robert J., et al. "Cannabidiol-Induced Apoptosis in Human Leukemia Cells: A Novel Role of Cannabidiol in the Regulation of p22phox and Nox4 expression." *Molecular Pharmacology* 70.3 (2006): 897–908.

McMeens, R.R. *Report of the Ohio State Medical Committee on Cannabis Indica: 1860, 15th Annual Meeting.*

McPartland, John M., et al. "Care and Feeding of the Endocannabinoid System: A Systematic Review of Potential Clinical Interventions That Upregulate the Endocannabinoid System." *PLoS One* 9.3 (2014): 1–81.

Mechoulam, Raphael. "Conversation with Raphael Mechoulam." *Addiction* (Abingdon, England) 2007: 887–893. http://onlinelibrary.wiley.com/doi/10.1111/j.1360-0443.2007. 01795.x/full.

_____. "Mechoulam on Cannabidiol: An Overview at the IACM Meeting in Cologne." *O'Shaughnessy's* Winter/Spring 2008: 1–2.

_____. "Mechoulam: The Relevance of the Receptor System Discovery. The Cannabis Rescheduling Petition." DrugScience.Org 2006.

_____, and L. Hanuš. "Cannabidiol: An Overview of Some Chemical and Pharmacological Aspects. Part I: Chemical Aspects." *Chemistry and Physics of Lipids* 121.1–2 (2002): 35–43.

_____, et al. "Cannabidiol: An Overview of Some Pharmacological Aspects." *The Journal of Clinical Pharmacology* (2002): 11S–19S.

_____. "Cannabidiol—Recent Advances." *Chemistry & Biodiversity* (2007): 1678–1692.

Mechoulam, R., and Y. Shvo. "Hashish I—The Structure of Cannabidiol." *Tetrahedron* 19.12 (1963): 2073–2078.

"Medical Marijuana and CBD Dosing." ProjectCBD.org.

"Medical Marijuana Doctors in Maine." Integr8Health.com.

Mikuriya, Tod. "Marijuana Medical Handbook." Draft. UK Cannabis Internet Activist—The Cannabis Information Site, 2006.

Miller, R.J. "The Cannabis Conundrum." *Proceedings of the National Academy of Science* 110.43 (2013): 1–2.

Mimeault, M., et al. "Anti-Proliferative and Apoptotic Effects of Anandamide in Human Prostatic Cancer Cell Lines: Implication of Epidermal Growth Factor Receptor Down-Regulation and Ceramide Production." *Prostate* 56.1 (2003): 1–12.

Monory, Krisztina, et al. "The Endocannabinoid System Controls Key Epileptogenic Circuits in the Hippocampus." *Neuron*, Aug. 17, 2006: 455–466.

Murphy, Kathleen. "How Marijuana Became Illegal: W.R. Hearst Pulled a Fast One on the American Medical Association." *Washington Free Press*, June 3, 2009. http://wafreepress. org/article/090304marijuana.shtml.

Naderi N., et al. "Evaluation of Interactions Between Cannabinoid Compounds and Diazepam in Electroshock-induced Seizure Model in Mice." *Journal of Neural Transmission* (2008): 1501–1511. http://www.ncbi.nlm.nih.gov/pubmed/18575801.

Naftali, T., et al. "Cannabis Induces a Clinical Response in Patients with Crohn's Disease: A Prospective Placebo-Controlled Study." *Clinical Gastroenterology and Hepatology* 11.10 (2013): 1276–1280.

Nagarkatti, P., et al. "Cannabinoids as Novel Anti-inflammatory Drugs." *Future Medicinal Chemistry* 1.7 (2009): 1333–1349.

National Institutes of Health. "NIDA Research on the Therapeutic Benefits of Cannabis and Cannabinoids." March 2014.

Notcutt, W., et al. "Initial Experiences with Medicinal Extracts of Cannabis for Chronic Pain: Results from 34 'N of 1' Studies." *Anaesthesia* 59.5 (2004): 440–452.

O'Brien, Charles P. "Drug Addiction and Drug Abuse." In *Goodman & Gilman's The Pharmacological Basis of Therapeutics*, Eleventh Ed., edited by Louis Goodman and Alfred Gilman, 607–627. New York: MacMillan, 2006.

Okura, Dan, et al. "The Endocannabinoid Anandamide Inhibits Voltage-Gated Sodium Channels Nav1. 2, Nav1. 6, Nav1. 7, and Nav1. 8 in Xenopus Oocytes." *Anesthesia & Analgesia* 118.3 (2014): 554–562.

Pacher, P., et al. "The Endocannabinoid System as an Emerging Target of Pharmacotherapy." *Pharmacology Reviews*, Sept. 2006, 58(3): 389–462.

Pate, David. "Taxonomy of Cannabinoids." In *Cannabis and Cannabinoids: Pharmacology, Toxicology, and Therapeutic Potential*, edited by Franjo Grotenhermen and Ethan Russo, 15–26. Binghamton, NY: Haworth Integrative Healing Press, 2002.

Pertwee, Roger. "Cannabinoid Pharmacology: The First 66 Years." *British Journal of Pharmacology* 141.S1 (2006): S163–S171.

Pertwee, R.G. "The Diverse CB1 and CB2 Receptor Pharmacology of Three Plant Cannabinoids: Delta9-tetrahydrocannabinol, Cannabidiol and Delta9-tetrahydrocannabivarin." *British Journal of Pharmacology* 153.2 (2008): 199–215.

Pertwee, R.G., et al. "Cannabinoid Receptors and Their Ligands: Beyond CB1 and CB2." *The American Society for Pharmacology and Experimental Therapeutics, Pharmacological Reviews* 62.4 (2010): 588–631.

_____, et al. "Spasticity and Chronic Pain." In *Cannabis in Medical Practice: A Legal, Historical and Pharmacological Overview of the Therapeutic Use of Marijuana*, edited by Mary Lynn Mathre, 112–124. Jefferson, NC: McFarland, 1997.

Phillips, David. "Marijuana Oil Brings Relief, Joy." Colorado Springs: *The Gazette*, December, 2013.

Platt, Michael. "Medical Marijuana Gives Epileptic Child New Lease on Life." TorontoSun.com, Apr. 26, 2014.

Porter, B.E., and C. Jacobson. "Report of a Parent Survey of Cannabidiol-Enriched Cannabis Use in Pediatric Treatment-Resistant Epilepsy." *Epilepsy & Behavior* 29.3 (2013): 574–577.

Powles, Thomas, et al. "Cannabis-induced Cytotoxicity in Leukemic Cell Lines: The Role of the Cannabinoid Receptors and the MAPK Pathway." *Blood* 105.3 (2005): 1214–1221.

Rabey, Steve. "Moraljuana." *The Gazette,* Colorado Springs, Feb. 9, 2014.

Rahn, Elizabeth J., and Andrea G. Hohmann. "Cannabinoids as Pharmacotherapies for Neuropathic Pain: From the Bench to the Bedside." Neurotherapeutics 6.4 (2009): 713–737.

Rajesh, M., et al. "Cannabidiol Attenuates Cardiac Dysfunction, Oxidative Stress, Fibrosis, and Inflammatory and Cell Death Signaling Pathways in Diabetic Cardiomyopathy." *Journal of the American College of Cardiology* 56.25 (2010): 2115–2125.

Ramer, Robert, et al. "Cannabidiol Inhibits Lung Cancer Cell Invasion and Metastasis via Intercellular Adhesion Molecule–1." *The FASEB Journal* 26.4 (2012): 1535–1548.

Randall, Robert C. "Glaucoma: A Patient's View." In *Cannabis in Medical Practice: A Legal, Historical and Pharmacological Overview of the Therapeutic Use of Marijuana,* edited by Mary Lynn Mathre, 94–111. Jefferson, NC: McFarland, 1997.

Rimmerman, N., et al. "Direct Modulation of the Outer Mitochondrial Membrane Channel, Voltage-Dependent Anion Channel 1 (VDAC1) by Cannabidiol: A Novel Mechanism for Cannabinoid-Induced Cell Death." *Cell Death & Disease,* Dec. 5, 2013: e949. http://www.ncbi.nlm.nih.gov/pmc/articles/PMC3877544/.

Roberts, P.J., and C.J. Der. "Targeting the Raf-MEK-ERK Mitogen-Activated Protein Kinase Cascade for the Treatment of Cancer." *Oncogene* 26.22 (2007): 3291–3310.

Rock, E.M., et al. "Evaluation of the Potential of the Phytocannabinoids, Cannabidivarin (CBDV) and Δ (9) -tetrahydrocannabivarin (THCV), to Produce CB1 Receptor Inverse Agonism Symptoms of Nausea in Rats." *British Journal of Pharmacology* 2013 170(3): 671–678.

Rodgers, Jakob. "A Growing Web for Relief." *The Gazette,* Colorado Springs, Dec. 4, 2014.

Roser, P., et al. "Potential Antipsychotic Properties of Central Cannabinoid (CB1) Receptor Antagonists." *World Journal of Biological Psychiatry* 11.2 (2010): 208–219.

Rucke, Katie. "Hemp Oil Versus CBD Oil: What's the Difference?" *Mint Press News,* 15 Jul. 2014.

Ruhaak, L.R., et al. "Evaluation of the Cyclooxygenase Inhibiting Effects of Six Major Cannabinoids Isolated from Cannabis Sativa." *Biological and Pharmaceutical Bulletin* 34.5 (2011): 774–778.

Russo, Ethan. "Cannabis Strains: Do Cannabis Strains Differ?" *International Association for Cannabinoid Medicines FAQ,* 24 Aug. 2014.

_____. "Clinical Endocannabinoid Deficiency (CECD): Can this Concept Explain Therapeutic Benefits of Cannabis in Migraine, Fibromyalgia, Irritable Bowel Syndrome and Other Treatment Related Conditions?" *Neuroendocrinology Letters* 29.2 (2008): 192–200.

_____, et al. "Phytochemical and Genetic Analyses of Ancient Cannabis from Central Asia." *Journal of Experimental Botany* 59.15 (2008): 4171–4182.

Sacco, Lisa, and Kristin Finklea. "State Marijuana Legalization Initiatives: Implications for Federal Law Enforcement." *Congressional Research Service Report for Congress,* Dec. 4, 2014.

Salazar, María, et al. "Cannabinoid Action Induces Autophagy-Mediated Cell Death Through Stimulation of ER Stress in Human Glioma Cells." *The Journal of Clinical Investigation* 119.5 (2009): 1359–1372.

"The Science of Medical Cannabis: A Conversation with Donald Abrams, M.D." YouTube.com, Oct. 14, 2010.

Scuderi, C., et al. "Cannabidiol Promotes Amyloid Precursor Protein Ubiquitination and Reduction of Beta Amyloid Expression in SHSY5YAPP+ Cells Through PPARγ Involvement." *Phytotherapy Research* 28.7 (2014): 1007–1013.

Seyfried, Thomas N., and Laura M. Shelton. "Cancer as a Metabolic Disease." *Nutrition & Metabolism* (Lond) 7.7 (2010): 269–270.

Sharkey, Keith. "The Endocannabinoid System and the Control of Gastrointestinal Function." eJournal, Dec. 2008.

Sherry, Amelia R. "Spotlight on Stearidonic Acid—Learn More About This Alternative Omega–3 Fatty Acid." Jul. 2014.

Shinjyo, N., and V. Di Marzo. "The Effect of Cannabichromene on Adult Neural Stem/Progenitor Cells." *Neurochemistry International* 63.5 (2013): 432–437.

Shrivastava, Ashutosh, et al. "Cannabidiol Induces Programmed Cell Death in Breast Cancer Cells by Coordinating the Cross-Talk Between Apoptosis and Autophagy." *Molecular Cancer Therapeutics* 10.7 (2011): 1161–1172.

Simpson, Rick. Personal Interview, 3 Sept. 2008.

Singh, Yadvinder, and Chamandeep Bali. "Cannabis Extract Treatment for Terminal Acute Lymphoblastic Leukemia with a Philadelphia Chromosome Mutation." *Case Reports in Oncology* 6.3 (2013): 585–592.

Smethurst, Annika. "Desperate Parents Turn to Medical Marijuana in Last-Ditch Effort to Improve Their Children's Lives." Heraldsun.com.au, Jan. 12, 2014.

Solinas, Marta, et al. "Cannabidiol, a Non-Psychoactive Cannabinoid Compound, Inhibits Proliferation and Invasion in U87-MG and T98G Glioma Cells Through a Multitarget Effect." *PloS One* 8.10 (2013): e76918.

Sosin, Daniel. "CDC Washington Testimony April 29 2014." CDC.gov, 29 Apr. 2014.

"Speaker." DavidBearmanMD.com.

Stanley, C.P., W.H. Hind, and S.E. O'Sullivan. "Is the Cardiovascular System a Therapeutic Target for Cannabidiol?" *British Journal of Clinical Pharmacology* 75.2 (2013): 313–322.

Starks, Michael. *Marijuana Chemistry: Genetics, Processing & Potency*. Berkeley, CA: Ronin Publishing, 1990.

"State Medical Marijuana Laws." *National Conference of State Legislatures*. Nov. 13, 2014. http://www.ncsl.org/research/health/state-medical-marijuana-laws.aspx.

Stewart, Kirsten. "Families Migrating to Colorado for a Medical Marijuana Miracle." *The Salt Lake Tribune*, Nov. 11, 2013. http://www.sltrib.com/sltrib/mobile3/57052556-219/piper-annie-seizures-cbd.html.csp.

Stingl, Jim. "Cannabis Oil's legalization in Wisconsin Too Late to Help 7-Year-Old Girl." *Journal Sentinel*, 13 May 2014. http://www.jsonline.com/news/milwaukee/7-year-old-face-of-fight-for-legalizing-cannabis-oil-dies-b99269328z1-259122301.html.

Suh, Dong H., et al. "Mitochondrial Permeability Transition Pore as a Selective Target for Anti-Cancer Therapy." *Frontiers in Oncology* 3.41 (2013).

Szalavitz, Maia. "Marijuana Compound Treats Schizophrenia with Few Side Effects: Clinical Trial." To,e/cp, Time Inc., 30 May 2012.

Taylor, Victoria. "Girl, 7, Who Became the Face of Legalizing Marijuana Oil in Wisconsin, Dies. *New York Daily News*, May 16, 2014.

Tetanish, Raissa. "Seized Marijuana Plants Had Value Up to $830,000: RCMP." Cumberland-NewsNow.com, Sept. 13, 2007.

_____. "Simpson Considers Leaving Country." CumberlandNewsNow.com, Feb. 11, 2008.

Torres, Marco. "Cannabis Oil Cures 8 Month Old Infant of Cancer, Dissolving Large Inoperable Tumor in 8 Months." PreventDisease.com, 24 Jun. 2014.

Turner, C.E., and M.A. ElSohly. "Biological Activity of Cannabichromene, Its Homologs and Isomers." *The Journal of Clinical Pharmacology* 21.8–9 (1981): 283S-291S.

"2014 Farm Bill—Section 7606" Vote Hemp Information, Aug. 28, 2014.

"U.N. Says U.S. Marijuana Legalization Violates International Law." *Newsweek*, 12 Nov. 2014.

Upton, R., et al., eds. *American Herbal Pharmacopoeia*. Scotts Valley, CA: American Herbal Pharmacopoeia, 2014.

"U.S. Federal Marijuana Farm to Offer New Strains." LeafScience.com, 25 Mar. 2014.

Vaccani, A., et al. "Cannabidiol Inhibits Human Glioma Cell Migration Through a Cannabinoid Receptor-Independent Mechanism." *British Journal of Pharmacology* 144.8 (2005): 1032–1036.

Valley, Jennifer. Stoney Girl Gardens Website, 1999.

Van Heerden, Adam. "Professor Raphael Mechoulam, the Father of Marijuana Research, Talks to NoCamels About His Studies and Breaking the Law in the Name of Science." NoCamels, Israeli Innovation News, Sept. 2013.

Van Klingeren, B., and M. Ten Ham. "Antibacterial Activity of Delta9-Tetrahydrocannabinol and Cannabidiol." *Antonie Van Leeuwenhoek* 42.1–2 (1976): 9–12.

Velasco, Guillermo, Cristina Sánchez, and Manuel Guzmán. "Towards the Use of Cannabinoids as Antitumour Agents." *Nature Reviews Cancer* 12.6 (2012): 436–444.

Wade, D.T., et al. "A Preliminary Controlled Study to Determine Whether Whole-Plant Cannabis Extracts Can Improve Intractable Neurogenic Symptoms." *Clinical Rehabilitation* 17.1 (2003): 21–29.

Wallace, Melisa, et al. "Assessment of the Role of CB1 Receptors in Cannabinoid Anticonvulsant Effects." *European Journal of Pharmacology*, Sept. 28, 2001: 51–57.

_____. "The Endogenous Cannabinoid System Regulates Seizure Frequency and Duration in a Model of Temporal Lobe Epilepsy." *Journal of Pharmacology and Experimental Therapeutics*, Oct. 2003: 129–137. http://www.ncbi.nlm.nih.gov/pubmed/12954810.

Walsh, S.K., et al. "Acute Administration of Cannabidiol in Vivo Suppresses Ischaemia-Induced Cardiac Arrhythmias and Reduces Infarct Size When Given at Reperfusion." *British Journal of Pharmacology* 160.5 (2010): 1234–1242.

Ward, Patrick S., and Craig B. Thompson. "Metabolic Reprogramming: A Cancer Hallmark Even Warburg Did Not Anticipate." *Cancer Cell* 21.3 (2012): 297–308.

Ware, Mark A., et al. "Smoked Cannabis for Chronic Neuropathic Pain: A Randomized Controlled Trial." *Canadian Medical Association Journal*, Aug. 30, 2010: E694–E701.

Wargent, E.T., et al. "The Cannabinoid Δ(9)-Tetrahydrocannabivarin (THCV) Ameliorates Insulin Sensitivity in Two Mouse Models of Obesity." *Nutrition & Diabetes* 27.3 (2013): e68.

Weed People Movie. WeedPeopleMovie.com.

Weiss, L., et al. "Cannabidiol Arrests Onset of Autoimmune Diabetes in NOD Mice." *Neuropharmacology* 54.1 (2008): 244–249.

_____. "Cannabidiol Lowers Incidence of Diabetes in Non-Obese Diabetic Mice." *Autoimmunity* 39.2 (2006): 143–151.

Welty, Timothy E., et al. "Cannabidiol: Promise and Pitfalls." *Epilepsy Currents* 14 (5) (201): 250–252.

Werz, Oliver, et al. "Cannflavins from Hemp Sprouts, a Novel Cannabinoid-Free Hemp Food Product, Target Microsomal Prostaglandin E_2 Synthase–1 and 5-Lipoxygenase." *PharmaNutrition* 2.3 (2014): 53–60.

"What Is Charas and How Do You Make It?" *Weed Street Journal*, 15 Jun. 2011.

Wild, David. "Pharmacy Practice News—Refractory CRPS Patients Discontinue Opiates with Cannabinoid Treatment." PharmacyPracticeNews.com. McMahon Publishing, 8 Feb. 2011.

Wilsey, Barth, et al. "Low-dose Vaporized Cannabis Significantly Improves Neuropathic Pain." *The Journal of Pain* 14.2 (2013): 136–148.

Wollstein, Jarret. "The Government's War on Property." *The Freeman: Foundation for Economic Education*. July 1, 1993.

Wyatt, Kristen. "State OKs $8 Mil in Marijuana Research." Colorado Springs: *The Gazette*, Dec. 18, 2014.

Young, Saundra. "Marijuana Stops Child's Severe Seizures." CNN.com, Aug. 7, 2013. http://www.cnn.com/2013/08/07/health/charlotte-child-medical-marijuana/index.html.

_____. "Medical Marijuana Research Stalls After Arizona Professor Is Let Go." *CNN Health News*, July 12, 2014.

Zeese, Kevin B. "Legal Issues Related to the Medical Use of Marijuana." In *Cannabis in Medical Practice: A Legal, Historical and Pharmacological Overview of the Therapeutic Use of Marijuana*, edited by Mary Lynn Mathre, 20–31. Jefferson, NC: McFarland.

Zhornitsky, S., and S. Potvin. "Cannabidiol in Humans—The Quest for Therapeutic Targets." *Pharmaceuticals* (Basel) 5.5 (2012): 529–552.

Zhu, HuiLing, et al. "Medicinal Compounds with Antiepileptic/Anticonvulsant Activities." *Epilepsia* 55.1, Jan. 2014: 3–16.

Zuardi, Antonio Waldo. "Cannabidiol: From an Inactive Cannabinoid to a Drug with Wide Spectrum of Action." *The Revista Brasileira de Psiquiatria* 30.3 (2008): 271–280.

_____, and Fracisco Guimães. "Cannabidiol as an Anxiolytic and Antipsychotic." In *Cannabis in Medical Practice: A Legal, Historical and Pharmacological Overview of the Therapeutic Use of Marijuana*, edited by Mary Lynn Mathre, 133–141. Jefferson, NC: McFarland, 1997.

_____, et al. "Cannabidiol, a Cannabis Sativa Constituent, as an Antipsychotic Drug." *Brazilian Journal of Medical and Biological Research* 39.4 (2006): 421–429.

_____. "Cannabidiol for the Treatment of Psychosis in Parkinson's Disease." *Journal of Psychopharmacology* (Oxford) 23.8 (2009): 979–983.

_____. "Cannabidiol Monotherapy for Treatment-Resistant Schizophrenia." *Journal of Psychopharmacology* (Oxford) 20.5 (2006): 683–686.

_____. "A Critical Review of the Antipsychotic Effects of Cannabidiol: 30 Years of a Translational Investigation." *Current Pharmaceutical Design* 18.32 (2012): 5131–5140.

Index

211